Paul J. Rajcok

LECTURES

in

NATUROPATHIC HYDROTHERAPY

by

Wade Boyle, N.D.

and

André Saine, N.D.

Buckeye Naturopathic Press
East Palestine, Ohio

Second Printing 1991

Third Printing 1993

ISBN O-9623518-1-4

Buckeye Naturopathic Press

E. Palestine, OH 44413

Dedicated to:

DRS. JOHN BASTYR
HAROLD DICK
and
LEO SCOTT

who have kept alive and nourished the tradition of constitutional hydrotherapy and passed it on to a new generation of naturopathic physicians.

ACKNOWLEDGEMENTS

The information in this book is based primarily on the teachings of three of Dr. O. G. Carroll's students, Drs. John Bastyr, Harold Dick, and Leo Scott, and his son, Dr. Bill Carroll, as well as the following works: *Rational Hydrotherapy* by John H. Kellogg; *Manual of Hydrotherapy and Massage* by Fred B. Moor, Stella C. Peterson, Ethel M. Manwell, Mary C. Noble and Gertrude Muench; *Home Remedies, Hydrotherapy, Massage, Charcoal and Other Simple Treatments* by Drs. Agatha and Calvin Thrash; *Nature Cure* by Henry Lindlahr; *My Water Cure* by Fr. Sebastian Kneipp; *An Epitome of Hydrotherapy* by Simon Baruch; and *Simple Water Treatments for the Home* by Charles Thomas et al. The valuable information from these sources is gratefully acknowledged.

We would also like to thank Drs. Francis Brinker, Joe Coletto, Leo Scott, Harold Dick, John Bastyr, Tori Hudson and Mr. Friedhelm Kirchfeld, Librarian of the National College of Naturopathic Medicine, for their valuable criticism of the manuscript. Mr. Kirchfeld deserves additional thanks for his help in obtaining research materials for the book.

PREFACE

This book is not a definitive text of hydrotherapy with exhaustive references and elaborate illustrations but rather a record of the lectures (rearranged here for the sake of continuity) presented by Dr. Saine or myself in the early 1980's at the National College of Naturopathic Medicine, John Bastyr College, and the Ontario College of Naturopathic Medicine. It is intended as a companion to personalized clinical instruction by qualified hydrotherapists and as a review and reference source for trained practitioners. It is *not* intended as a *course in itself* in hydrotherapy. This is especially true in regards to the constitutional treatment of Dr. O. G. Carroll. While the basics of this treatment are outlined in detail, its clinical use should not be undertaken without prior instruction by qualified personnel in a clinical setting.

A number of excellent texts on hydrotherapy already exist. Some of them, as previously acknowledged, provided the basis for many of these lectures. However, few of these books are specifically oriented toward naturopathic practice, and, of course, none of them deal with Dr. Carroll's constitutional treatment. Although, due to limited resources, a number of shortcomings are built into this first edition, it is hoped that, despite imperfections, its emphasis on these neglected aspects of hydrotherapy will justify its appearance. For the sake of improving future editions the comments, corrections and suggestions of its readers are sincerely solicited.

Wade Boyle, N.D.
East Palestine, Ohio 1988

CONTENTS

Acknowledgements v
Preface ii

I.
BASIC PRINCIPLES

1. Introduction 3
2. Modern History of Hydrotherapy 5
3. Philosophy of Naturopathic Hydrotherapy 17
4. Terminology 19
5. Properties of Water 23
6. Properties of Hot and Cold 29
7. Principles of Circulation 35
8. Manipulation of Circulation by Hot and Cold 41
9. Principles of Hydrotherapy 47
10. Fever and Naturopathic Hydrotherapy 53

II.
DEMONSTRATIONS

11. Introduction - Hydrotherapy Equipment and Temperature Conversions 65
12. Hot Foot Bath 69
13. Russian Bath 73
14. Heating Compresses 77
15. Steam Inhalation 83
16. Sitz Bath 87
17. Fomentations 91
18. Neutral Bath 95
19. Ice Pack 99
20. Enemas 103
21. Salt Glow 107
22. Alternate Baths 111

23. Poultices........ 115
24. *Blitz Guss*........ 119
25. Wet Sheet Pack........ 123
26. Cold Mitten Friction........ 129

III.
CONSTITUTIONAL APPROACH

27. Demonstration of Constitutional Treatment........ 135
28. Auscultation........ 147
29. Hydrotherapy and Electrotherapy........ 153
30. Hydrotherapy and Botanical Medicine........ 157
31. Hydrotherapy and Nutrition........ 167
32. Healing Crisis........ 175
33. Management of Acute Disease........ 187
34. Management of Chronic Disease........ 205
35. Constitutional Hydrotherapy in Office Practice........ 211
36. Conclusion........ 219

Bibliography........ 221
Index........ 227

I.
BASIC PRINCIPLES

1. COURSE INTRODUCTION

> "No remedy in the entire materia medica demands as clear judgement and as much knowledge of the patient's condition as does the application of water."
>
> — Simon Baruch

The goal of this course of lectures is to present the basic principles of naturopathic hydrotherapy, not so they may be memorized by the student but so they may be understood. The hallmark of any naturopathic treatment is that it is individually suited to each patient. It is impossible to custom-tailor any treatment to a given patient without a thorough knowledge of the principles underlying that treatment. This is as true for hydrotherapy as it is for homeopathy, acupuncture or any other modality.

There are many variables in hydrotherapy. Some, such as the temperature, duration and extent of the treatment, are under the direct control of the hydrotherapist, while others, such as the patient's disease, vitality and ability to tolerate hydrotherapy, are totally outside of the hydrotherapist's control. The successful hydrotherapist must manipulate the variables under his control to create a treatment which matches as closely as possible the picture presented by the variables outside his control. The ability to do this is based not on memorization but on understanding.

In this spirit the presentations which follow will emphasize the most basic principles of hydrotherapy, sometimes in a repetitive manner. The intent here is not to insult anyone's intelligence but rather to insure that everyone has an adequate chance to come to a thorough and lasting understanding of the theoretical basis of hydrotherapy so that he or she will be able to use hydrotherapy confidently, frequently and successfully.

After we cover the basic principles, we will begin instruction in the various water treatments. While we will spend ample time demonstrating the exact procedures and explaining indications and contraindications, we will take special pains to emphasize the mechanism by which each treatment achieves its effects. A mechanism is the practical heart of a principle. The student must understand the mechanism of each treatment, first, so he or she can adapt the treatment to each patient's needs, and second, so he or she can give a credible explanation of the treatment to the patient. Hydrotherapy, like some other natural modalities, has a public relations problem with certain patients. Many patients rightfully want to know how and why a treatment works. When you get into the complexities of homeopathy or acupuncture, most patients are willing to take your word for it if the concepts go beyond their abilities to comprehend. But they figure they should be able to understand something as simple as water. So it is important for the hydrotherapist to be able to give accurate and convincing explanations of treatments, especially those involving procedures, such as applying cold, wet towels to the chest or cold, wet socks to the feet, which might seem odd or even silly to the patient without an understanding of their physiological effects. Earning the patient's confidence and compliance with intelligent answers to his questions is an important part of the art of medicine.

Once we have mastered the principles, mechanisms and procedures of the various hydrotherapy treatments, we will then attempt to integrate hydrotherapy into a comprehensive approach to a wide variety of medical conditions both acute and chronic. Naturopathic hydrotherapy is, by definition, hydrotherapy which is readily joined to other natural modalities, such as nutrition, herbs and homeopathy, to enhance the patient's ability to achieve better health.

Before we commence, let's consider the history of hydrotherapy.

2. MODERN HISTORY OF HYDROTHERAPY

> "While other professions and trades regard the study of the history of their subject as an important element in their education, the physician alone permits this profitable field to remain uncultivated."
>
> — Simon Baruch

The modern history of hydrotherapy is a tangle of overlapping influences among orthodox medical doctors, untrained empirics and trained but unorthodox medical practitioners. John Floyer (1649-1734), a Litchfield, England physician who advocated cold bathing, is perhaps the best figure with whom to start. His book, *The History of Hot and Cold Bathing,* first appeared in 1697 and went through six editions. It was translated into German in 1749 and is presumed to have influenced Johann S. Hahn (1696-1773), who, along with his father and brother, established the principles of modern hydrotherapy in Germany, applying it successfully in both acute and chronic diseases, especially smallpox.

The Hahns lived and practiced in the part of Austria known as Silesia. While no direct connection has been uncovered, it seems likely that the work of these medical doctors provided at least an indirect influence upon Vincent Priessnitz (1799-1852), the unschooled peasant of Graefenberg, Silesia who achieved spectacular success with water treatments. As a boy on his father's farm Priessnitz noticed how animal sprains, bruises and tumors healed more quickly when bathed with cold water. An elderly neighbor who treated cattle with water taught the art to the young Priessnitz who used it with success on a number of animals. In 1816 at the age of seventeen Priessnitz was injured in a farm accident and broke two ribs. When the surgeon he consulted said he could not help, Priessnitz reduced the fractures himself by pressing his rib cage against a chair; then he kept his chest wrapped in a cold towel and drank plenty of cold water. Within a few days he had regained his health.

Priessnitz was soon treating his neighbors with cold water. Experiments he performed convinced him that sweating treatments combined with cold water treatments worked even better in cases such as gout and rheumatism. His success was such that his house soon became too small to hold all those who came for help. Priessnitz had no formal medical training, but in 1830 the Austrian government gave him special authorization to treat patients by his own unique methods. Demand for Priessnitz' water cure became so great that the government was forced to build new roads to facilitate access to his establishment. In 1840 he treated nearly 1600 patients from all over the world using primarily cold water treatments and simple diet. Physicians from many countries made pilgrimages to Priessnitz' mountain home and left to establish institutions modelled on his. Despite the previous advocacy of many respected medical men, water treatment did not become widely used until it was popularized by Priessnitz, the Silesian farm boy.

As we shall see shortly, Priessnitz had a profound influence upon the development of water cure in America. But his influence was just as important in Austria and Germany. One of his most able students was J.H. Rausse (1805-1848) who wrote *The Water Cure Applied to Every Known Disease.* Rausse later published a work entitled *Errors of Physicians and Others in the Practice of Water Cure* under the name Francke wherein he respectfully criticized some of Priessnitz' harsher water-cure methods and emphasized the need to individualize the treatments to the needs and tolerances of the patients. With considerable insight he stated, "Priessnitz is the discover(er) and hero of hydrotherapy; but he is not its master and finisher."

Others following Priessnitz were Johann Schroth (1798-1856) who combined dry fasting and sweat baths with water treatments; Louis Kuhne (1834-1907), whose book, *Neo-Naturopathy,* articulated his

"Unity of Disease" theory; Adolphe Just (1859-1939?) who wrote *Return to Nature;* and F. E. Bilz (1842-1922) whose book, *The Natural Healing Method,* became a nature cure classic. But the most successful and influential water curist after Priessnitz was Father Kneipp.

When he initially applied for the priesthood, Sebastian Kneipp (1821-1897) was rejected, because he had tuberculosis. After curing himself of his disease by the use of water treatments and diet, he was admitted to the priesthood and he began to treat his sick parishoners by the methods which had benefited him. His rise to international prominence as a lay healer paralleled that of Priessnitz several decades earlier. His book, *My Water Cure,* in which he detailed his water and herb treatments and advocated barefoot walking in dew and snow, went through many editions and translations. As we shall see shortly, he had a very strong and direct influence upon the development of hydrotherapy and naturopathy in the United States. But first, let's go back to England and John Floyer again.

The peasantry of all countries seem to have been more familiar with the therapeutic virtues of water than most trained physicians. This was no less true in England where Dr. Floyer published his influential work, than in other countries. In 1747 John Wesley (1703-1791), the founder of Methodism and a minister rather than a doctor, published *Primitive Physick,* a compilation of useful folk remedies, many of them employing water applications.

In 1752 Tobias Smollet (1721-1771), the English surgeon and novelist, published his "Essay on the External Use of Water." In 1797 another British physician, James Currie (1756-1805) published his study on the use of water in treating febrile illnesses. His work, which was the first to insist on thermometric monitoring of fever patients as a guide to water treatment, had an impact in America where he also practiced.

Next came James Gully (1808-1883) whose 1846 book, *The Water Cure in Chronic Disease,* was influential not only in England but also in France where Louis Fleury (1815-1872) would six years later publish his *Traite-Pratique et Raisonne D'Hydrotherapie* which put the cold douche on scientific footing as a medical therapy. With the help of other French physicians, the emerging medical science of hydrotherapy spread to the medical academies of Austria, the country already famous for the use of water cures by untrained laymen. Most prominent among the Viennese water physicians was Wilhelm Winternitz (1834-1912). He wrote over 200 articles and books on hydrotherapy, trained hundreds of doctors and nurses in his techniques and treated thousands of patients at his Kaltenleutgeben institutes. He was the first to bring out the most important physiological truth about hydrotherapy — that its strongest effects are mediated through the nervous system. He was personal friend and mentor to Drs. Simon Baruch and John Harvey Kellogg who successfully brought Winternitz' scientific hydrotherapeutics to the United States.

John Harvey Kellogg (1852-1943) helped establish and run the famous Battle Creek Sanitorium in Michigan where he employed numerous types of water treatments and conducted experiments on the effects of different applications. His monumental work, *Rational Hydrotherapy,* first appeared in 1901 and remains to this day the definitive textbook of hydrotherapy. Kellogg was a voluminous and able writer, and his works on massage, sine wave and diet remain classics in their fields.

Simon Baruch's (1840-1921) goal in life was to separate scientific hydrotherapy from the water cure employed by empirics and to establish it as an acceptable part of orthodox medicine. After studying with Winternitz, he returned to the United States and practiced hydrotherapy successfully on a hospital-wide scale. He documented thousands of serious cases treated by water, and his books, *The Principles and Practice of Hydrotherapy* (1898) and *An Eptitome of Hydrotherapy* (1920), are among the most valuable in the literature. While he had a temporary impact on medical care in New York state where he practiced, in the end his valiant efforts failed to win his orthodox colleagues over to his favorite treatment. Baruch would, no doubt, be uncomfortable being included in this history. He probably would regard us naturopaths as he did the empirics of his day — that is, with mixed emotions. He would disdain us for being "irregulars" but he would be grudgingly grateful to us for studying and employing the hydrotherapy which he loved so much.

Having briefly traced the modern origins of hydrotherapy in England

and on the continent, let's return to the early eighteenth century and look at hydrotherapy's development in America. In 1725 John Smith, who was undoubtedly aware of the work of Floyer, wrote *The Curiosities of Common Water . . . in Curing Cholera, Intemperance and Other Maladies,* the first known American work. Later in the century Benjamin Rush (1745-1813), one of the most distinguished physicians in the young country, used cold water and ice successfully in his Philadelphia practice while Drs. Bard and Hosack did similar work at New York Hospital. In 1850 Dr. John Bell (1796-1872) published his *Treatise on Baths* which stood as the most authoritative work in English until Winternitz' writings were translated 30 years later. John Harvey Kellogg was well aware of Bell's work and acknowledged its value.

While these respected, orthodox practitioners contributed to the growth of hydrotherapy in America, there were a number of irregular practitioners who embraced hydrotherapy and brought it to even greater prominence. They were among the many practitioners who journeyed to Graefenberg, Silesia to witness and experience the work of Priessnitz. They called the system they brought back to the United States hydropathy or water cure.

The first great wave of hydropathy in America, came in the 1840's. Robert Wesselhoeft (1796-1852), a German who had been cured of rheumatic fever by Priessnitz, and his brother, William, immigrated to America, undertook medical studies and eventually set up a water-cure establishment in Vermont based on the practices of Priessnitz. Incorporated in 1845 as the Brattleboro Infirmary, it became the most exclusive water cure in the country, counting such luminaries as Henry Wadsworth Longfellow and Harriet Beecher Stowe among its patrons. It should be mentioned that the Wesselhoefts knew Samuel Hahnemann (1755-1843), the founder of homeopathy, in Germany and were influenced by his beliefs, not only concerning homeotherapeutics but also about water treatments. It appears that Hahnemann was well acquainted with the work of the Drs. Hahn mentioned earlier. David Ruggles (1810-1849), a patient and later student of the Wesselhoefts, is noteworthy as one of the few blacks in the hydropathic movement. He was very active in the Underground Railroad and treated such famous abolitionists as Sojourner Truth, William Lloyd Garrison, and John Brown's mother, Mary, with hydropathy. An 1849 editorial in the Boston *Liberator* referred to him as the "Priessnitz of America."

About the same time the Wesselhoefts and Ruggles became active in this country, Joel Shew (1816-1855) began the publication of *The Water Cure Journal* which, within a few years, achieved a circulation in excess of 50,000 copies. He had been a daguerreotyper and became an invalid from overexposure to the mercury, iodine and bromine compounds with which he worked. He made two trips to Graefenberg and regained sufficient health to become one of the most indefatigable proponents of the water cure. He dedicated his 1847 *Water-Cure Manual* "To the Immortal Priessnitz." In 1844 his wife, Mary Louis Shew, published *Water-Cure for Ladies.*

Shew's most notable associate was Russell Thatcher Trall (1812-1877) who established a water-cure house in New York City as early as 1844. He collaborated with Shew on various health publications and water cure projects. He wrote over 25 books, the most famous being his *Hydropathic Encyclopedia* which appeared in 1852. He was a follower of the hygienic reforms of Sylvester Graham, and, while he acknowledged his debt to Graham and Priessnitz, he claimed to have improved on both. In the late 1850's he set up the Hygeio-Therapeutic College in New York City which included instruction in medicine, electricity, Swedish movement, gymnastics, diet and water treatment in its curriculum. The selection of the name Hygeio-Therapy was an attempt on Trall's part to separate himself from the more radical hydropathists who claimed all disease could be cured by cold water alone. The question of respectability was and always will be central to medicine. It is an interesting sidelight that while Trall tried to distance himself from his less respectable hydropathic colleagues, John Harvey Kellogg took pains to distance himself from Trall whose school he had studied at when he first took up medicine. Nowhere in Kellogg's subsequent career did he acknowledge any connection with the less orthodox Dr. Trall.

To complete this picture of hydropathy in mid-nineteenth century America, mention should be made of J. H. Pulte (1811-1884) and H. P. Gatchell (1815-1889), two Ohio homeopaths who published the

American Magazine of Homeopathy and Hydropathy in the 1850's. Also of note are Mary Gove Nichols (1810-1884), a women's rights and health reformer, who began treating her neighbors with cold water as early as 1832. She became a patient and student of the Wesselhoefts and Shew. In 1851 she and her husband, Thomas Low Nichols (1816-1901), founded the American Hydropathic Institute in New York, a coeducational medical school which they claimed was the first in the world based on water-cure principles. It is a significant social and medical fact that two-thirds of the patients at the Wesselhoefts' Brattleboro water cure were women — this in an era when women were discouraged from travel. Women were drawn to hydropathy because the water treatments were effective and were usually conducted in an atmosphere of freely given information concerning female health problems which was hard to come by elsewhere.

In the last quarter of the nineteenth century the popularity of hydropathy in general declined. However, the principles and practices were maintained and advanced by James Caleb Jackson (1814-1895). He treated thousands of patients with, he claimed, 95% success at his institute called "Our Home on the Hillside" in Dansville, New York. He believed that water treatments were most effective when combined with other hygienic measures. He employed fresh air, simple foods, water, sunlight, dress, exercise, sleep, rest, social influence and mental and moral forces in a system he termed "Psycho-Hygienic." His 1874 book, *How to Treat the Sick Without Medicine,* articulates his beliefs and experience and is well worth reading today. Another interesting sidelight: Jackson published an article in the Yates County *Chronicle* in 1863 on diptheria which introduced Ellen G. White (1827-1915), the founder of Seventh Day Adventism, to hydrotherapy; and it was Mrs. White who later sponsored the work of John Harvey Kellogg, one of the most important figures in the modern history of hydrotherapy.

We have brought the developments in hydrotherapy in England, on the continent and in the United States roughly up to the end of the nineteenth century. We have seen the hydrotherapeutic and hygienic basis for naturopathy. Now, with the work of Benedict Lust and Henry Lindlahr, naturopathy, and, therefore, naturopathic hydrotherapy, come into being.

Benedict Lust (1872-1943) was born in Germany and contracted TB in his youth. As a last resort he went to Father Kneipp who restored him to health. In 1892 he was commissioned by Kneipp to introduce the Kneipp water cure in the United States. This Lust did with great success and added to it chiropractic, massage and other emerging natural therapies. In 1896 he founded the American Naturopathic Association and began publishing the first of his many natural health journals. He was a tireless, partisan promoter of naturopathy and was greatly pleased when a regular medical publication referred to him as "the greatest menace to official medicine."

The other pillar of naturopathy is Henry Lindlahr (1852-1925). In 1893 he was a real estate tycoon — the mayor, banker and leading citizen of Kalispell, Montana. At 41 years of age, in the prime of his life, he weighed over 250 pounds and soon found out he had diabetes mellitus. Having been advised by the best American doctors to settle his affairs, he journeyed to Vienna to consult the most learned European authorities and was told the same thing. A friend prevailed on him to visit Father Kneipp who smelled Lindlahr's breath, looked at his obese frame and said, "You have the sugar disease. You are a pig. You will take sitz baths, live on fruits and greens and vegetables alone. You shall have no breads, no cereals, no meats." By spring of the next year Lindlahr was free of sugar and, in a few more months, had lost over 40 pounds and was in excellent health. Grateful for his reprieve, he visited other European health centers and studied their methods of natural healing. He returned to the United States, took up the formal study of medicine and eventually established a sanitarium in Chicago which had one of the most advanced diagnostic departments of any medical facility in the country. There he treated hundreds of patients each day by the natural methods he had learned and developed. The basement of his sanitarium contained extensive hydrotherapeutic installations. His 1913 book, *Nature Cure,* is absolutely must reading for anyone who wants to practice naturopathic hydrotherapy or any other naturopathic therapy.

Others who studied with Kneipp and brought his water cure practices to the United States were Father Rougé who headed the Mt. Carmel Orphan Asylum in New Orleans in the 1890's and published a book in 1903 recounting the cures of 85 patients by the Kneipp method; Alex LeDoux, a medical doctor who studied with Kneipp and founded the LeDoux Institute of Natural Therapy in New Orleans in 1895; and Henry Lahn, another student of Kneipp's whose book, *Diagnosis from the Eye,* published in the late 1890's, was the first iridology text in English. It also contained a chapter on natural healing methods including hydrotherapy.

This brings us to the primary objective of this history, Dr. O. G. Carroll (1879-1962). The centerpiece of this course is Dr. Carroll's constitutional hydrotherapy treatment. He is, therefore, the central character in this historical sketch. He was born in Missouri. As a child he was afflicted with rheumatic fever and juvenile arthritis. He was cured of these problems by Dr. LeDoux and stayed on at LeDoux's institute to study his methods. Later, he preceptored with an old-time Thomsonian doctor who taught him the use of herbs. He studied at the Cleveland Chiropractic College in Chicago and, while in that city, practiced and studied with Lindlahr and Lahn for four years. In 1908 he moved to Spokane, Washington and became one of the first naturopathic practitioners in the west. In 1917 he established his sanitarium in Spokane which ran continuously until his death in 1962. He was the busiest health practitioner of any persuasion in the United States in the 1930's and 40's. His practice centered around the constitutional treatment which he had perfected by 1923 and which did not change for the next 40 years. Dr. Carroll was a fearless practitioner and never shied away from even the toughest, most hopeless cases. At various points he treated both Lindlahr and Lust. He cured Kellogg's wife of asthma. Dr. Carroll's work would be lost to us but for the efforts of several doctors who worked and studied with him.

Dr. John Bastyr, probably the greatest living naturopath, had established a busy practice by 1940 in Seattle. After referring several very difficult cases to Dr. Carroll, who promptly cured them, Dr. Bastyr decided to close his practice and go to Spokane and study with Dr. Carroll. After six months with Dr. Carroll, Dr. Bastyr resumed his practice in Seattle, where he continues to this day to integrate his own version of the constitutional treatment with other naturopathic therapies.

One of the greatest living naturopathic hydrotherapist is Dr. Harold Dick of Spokane, Washington. He was an auto mechanic in Boise, Idaho when the life of his hopelessly sick brother was saved by a single 400-mile car trip to visit Dr. Carroll. Impressed by the power of Dr. Carroll's treatments, Harold Dick undertook formal naturopathic training and then spent three years (1955-1958) with Dr. Carroll. Since it is impossible to do justice to Dr. Dick's colorful account of his experiences with Dr. Carroll, we urge all of you to view the videotapes of Dr. Dick on file at the library of the National College of Naturopathic Medicine in Portland, Oregon for yourselves.

One of the patients of Dr. Carroll's during Dr. Bastyr's stay with him was a very sick young man of 20 named Leo Scott who had visited 10 other doctors to no avail. Eventually cured by Dr. Carroll, he was inspired to take up naturopathic medical studies, and, having completed them, worked with Dr. Carroll from 1958-1962.

Both Dr. Scott and Dr. Dick maintain practices in Spokane. It is through the work of Drs. Bastyr, Dick and Scott and Dr. Bill Carroll, O. G.'s son who practiced at the sanitarium with his father for 20 years, that Dr. Carroll's work has been preserved for this new generation of naturopathic hydrotherapists.

In summary, we can see that modern hydrotherapy originated in Europe and that two major waves of influence, one in the middle of the nineteenth century and the other at the end of the nineteenth century, brought it to America. Out of all this historical information we have presented, what is important for you, as students, to remember? You must know Priessnitz and Kneipp; their work is the original basis for naturopathy. You must know Winternitz, Baruch and Kellogg; they put hydrotherapy on a scientific footing. You must know Lust and Lindlahr, the two true fathers of naturopathy. And, of course you must know Drs. Carroll, Bastyr, Dick and Scott whose recent work you are inheriting.

A flow chart sketching out the prominent historical figures follows.

MODERN HYDROTHERAPY HISTORICAL FLOW CHART
(Lines represent direct or indirect influence)

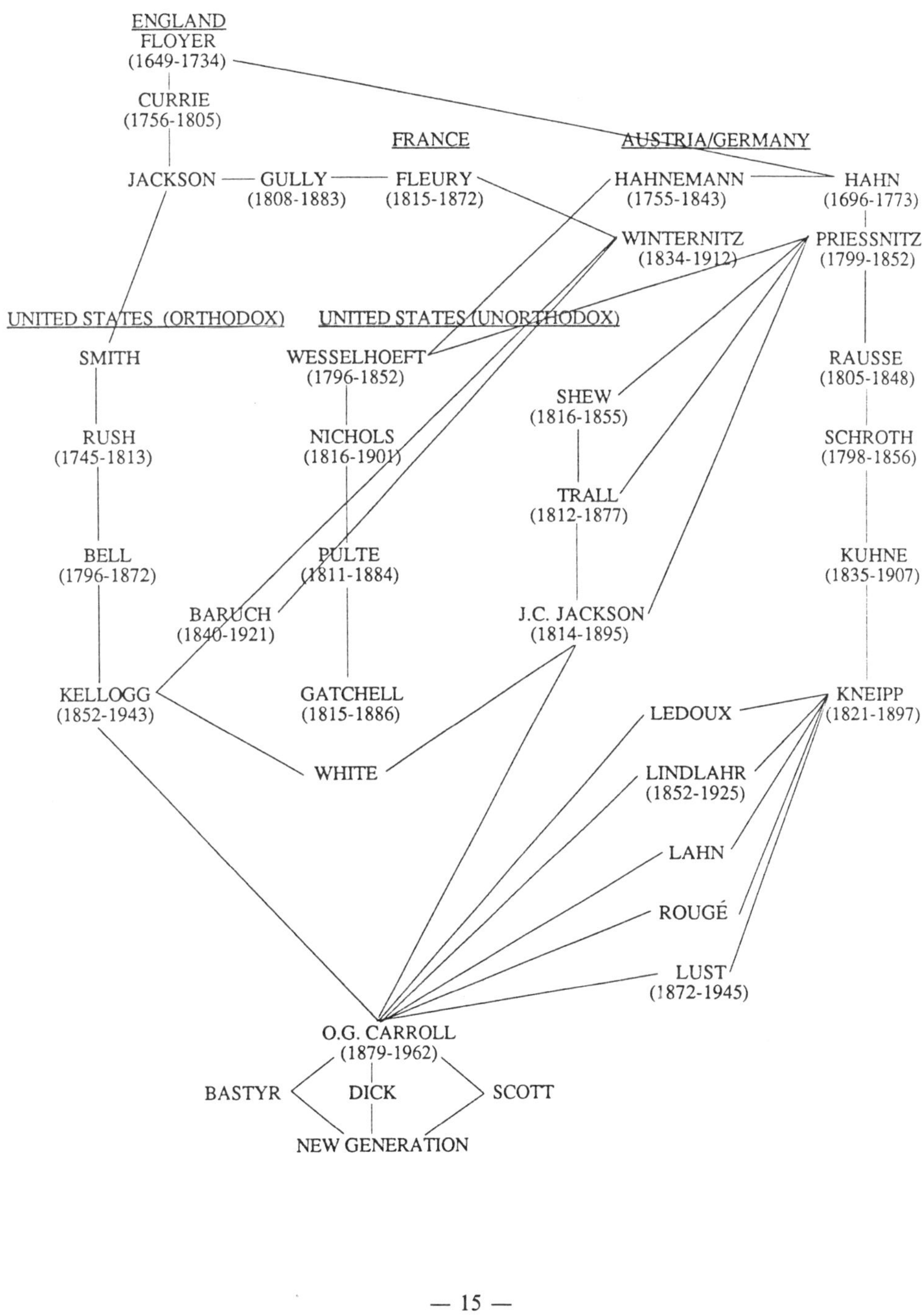

3. PHILOSOPHY OF NATUROPATHIC HYDROTHERAPY

> "Our job is to make over the blood. Until we do, we're just spinning our wheels."
>
> — Harold Dick

Once we embark on the practical study of naturopathic hydrotherapy, the philosophy underlying this modality will be gradually revealed and then frequently repeated. But to make sure no one misses it, let us state it clearly and simply from the outset.

The working hypothesis of naturopathic hydrotherapy is that health, and therefore healing, is proportional to normal flow of healthy blood. Specifically, this refers to the quantity and the quality of blood flowing through a given tissue. The hydrotherapist seeks to normalize the quantity of blood circulating through a given area during a given period of time. In some cases this will mean an increase in circulation and in other cases a reduction. In all cases the hydrotherapist seeks to improve the quality of blood in circulation.

This is where naturopathic hydrotherapy departs from conventional hydrotherapy. Medical doctors and physical therapists recognize the mechanical effects of water temperature on circulation, e.g., that hot water will help relax a tight muscle or that an ice pack can limit the swelling of a sprained ankle, but that is as far as they go. Naturopathic hydrotherapists, while making ready use of such mechanical circulatory effects, also believe that water treatments can affect the quality of blood in circulation. It is a notion, unique to naturopathic medicine, that by enhancing blood flow through the organs of elimination, such as the skin, liver, kidney and bowels, detoxification, and thereby improvement, of the blood takes place. In addition to improving blood by eliminating undesirable elements such as waste products, naturopathic hydrotherapists believe that water treatments can also help build the blood up by increasing desirable elements such as oxygen, nutrients, red cells, and white cells, etc. This is done primarily through treatments which tonify the digestive organs and thereby improve the nutrition received by the blood.

The naturopathic hydrotherapist views blood as the conveyer of life. As will be seen, hydrotherapy is the manipulation of circulation to maximize the life-giving properties of blood. Naturopathic hydrotherapy works because it optimizes the quality of blood while improving the efficiency of its circulation.

4. TERMINOLOGY

To some extent hydrotherapy has its own peculiar language. What follows is not an exhaustive list of all the terms used in hydrotherapy, but an introduction to the most important ones, grouped loosely according to topic rather than listed alphabetically. Certain of these terms are defined in contradictory ways by various authorities; therefore, liberties have been taken with these few terms to make them consistent in their meanings and, therefore, more useful for our purposes.

Hydrotherapy: the application of water in any form, either externally or internally, in the treatment of disease and the maintenance of health.

Hydropathy: refers to the "water cure" which arose from the empirical tradition and professed to cure all diseases by use of water, especially cold water.

Balneology or balneotherapy: the science of baths and their therapeutic uses.

Crenology or crenotherapy: therapeutic use of waters from mineral springs.

(Note: the previous two definitions are included as a point of interest but will not figure directly into the course material.)

Ablution: application of water by the hand which may be covered with a bath mitt or towel.

Affusion: the pouring of water in a stream on the body or part of the body. Usually used to lower body temperature in fever.

Douche: a stream of water directed against a part of the body or into a body cavity.

Clyster: a fluid injection into the rectum; an enema.

Poultice: a soft, moist mass spread between layers of cloth and applied hot to a given area in order to create moist local heat or counterirritation, e.g., a mustard plaster. Also called a cataplasm.

Compress: a pad of moist folded linen or other material applied with pressure; it is sometimes medicated.

Heating compress: a mild application of moist heat for several hours by means of a cold compress applied to a part and covered with dry flannel which allows the compress to be warmed by the circulation it stimulates. *Note:* this term causes more confusion than any other in hydrotherapy, so let's spend a moment to understand it. A heating compress is *not* a hot compress. A heating compress is a *cold* compress which becomes heated by the body part to which it is applied. You must grasp this important distinction to communicate reliably with other hydrotherapists.

Fomentation: a very hot, moist application, usually made of wool; it is sometimes medicated. Also called a stupe.

Derivation: the drawing of blood or lymph from one part of the body by increasing the amount of blood or lymph to another part.

Retrostasis: the driving of blood or lymph from one area of the body to another area.

Alternate: a series of alternating hot and cold applications to the same body area consisting of at least three applications of each, the duration of the cold applications being approximately one-fourth to one-half as long as the hot applications.

Revulsive: a single prolonged application of heat followed by a single brief application of cold. (Note: These previous two terms are frequently used interchangeably, and it is not crucial to be strict in distinguishing them).

Fluxion: a great increase in the rapidity of the blood current in a particular body part; active or arterial hyperemia.

Depletion: reduction of blood in a congested area, usually by prolonged cold applications.

Other terms will arise, and we will define them as we go along. These we have just gone over are the most basic, and we will have frequent cause to refer back to them.

5. PROPERTIES OF WATER

> "No remedial agent merits the confidence of the physician unless it fulfills the following conditions: (a) ready accessibility; (b) a rationale ascertained by experiments on a physiologic basis; (c) facility of dosage; (d) reliable clinical observations . . . Water meets all these demands . . . Water is not only readily accessible, but it may be used in the liquid, solid and vaporized form, each of which has its therapeutic value."
>
> — Simon Baruch

Before discussing the properties of water relevant to hydrotherapy, there are two introductory points we should make. The first concerns the "secret" of hydrotherapy and the second involves a warning about hydrotherapy's proper use.

If you are going to be hydrotherapists, it is only fair that we let you in on the secret of hydrotherapy from the outset which is that, aside from its universal solvent action, water possesses no innate healing qualities. If it did, there would not be so many sick people in the world. In fact, the term "hydrotherapy" is, in some ways, a misnomer and should more properly be called "thermotherapy," i.e., the treatment of disease by the application of hot and cold. We know that therapeutic heat may be applied to the body by various methods, e.g., the heating pad or the infrared lamp, but one of the most efficacious ways is by water. By convention we use the term "hydrotherapy" to describe these applications of hot (and cold) via water. But it should be remembered that the primary value of water in healing is its ability to carry heat. In hydrotherapeutics water is the medium and heat (or cold) is the message. To summarize this in strictly naturopathic terms: neither water nor heat nor cold heals; only the body heals; but hot and cold via water can enhance the capacity of the body to heal. (We use the terms "hot" and "heat" interchangeably; while not proper diction, it is common parlance among hydrotherapists.)

The introductory warning is this. Heat and water are low on the list of therapeutic prestige not only in orthodox circles but in naturopathic circles as well. While their usefulness in certain limited situations is acknowledged, their powerfulness rarely is. But heat and water are two of the most potent therapeutic agents available to any healer. If water were not of central importance to health, the body would not be made of such a large percentage of it; if heat were not vitally important to health, the body would not be equipped to maintain such a narrow thermic range. Homeopathy, acupuncture and allopathic drugs constitute powerful modalities which must be used with accuracy and precision. We want to impress upon you that water treatments belong in the same category. We want you to overcome any prejudices you may have about the ordinariness of water and heat so that you will use them in your practice, so that you can convince your patients to submit to them, and so that you will not hurt someone by applying them in a sloppy or inappropriate fashion. Water and heat are potent modalities which must be used with care and respect. Applied properly they can do much good; applied improperly they can do much harm. In the words of Dr. Baruch: "No remedy in the entire materia medica demands as clear judgement and as much knowledge of the patient's condition as does the application of water."

Now on to our main topic, the properties of water.

We will not catalogue all the virtues of water, but we do want to review the most basic properties of water pertinent to hydrotherapy. Besides its obvious abundance, affordability, availability, and the ease with which its temperature and pressure may be measured and controlled, there are three practical qualities of water we want to emphasize.

First and most important is the ability of water to absorb and give off large quantities of heat. From your general chemistry you will remember the term, "specific heat." Specific heat is the number of calories required to raise the temperature of one gram of a substance one degree centigrade. Every substance has its own specific heat. Water has one of the highest specific heats — approximately ten times higher than iron and approximately 30 times higher than lead or mercury. In fact, the specific heat of water is the standard against which the specific heats of other substances are measured. The significance of this in terms of hydrotherapy is that it takes a lot of heat to raise the temperature of water, and therefore, when it cools, water gives off a lot of heat. This makes water an excellent vehicle for carrying heat. Thus any hydrotherapeutic measure, such as Dr. Carroll's constitutional treatment, which uses water in its liquid state, derives much of its therapeutic power from the heat-absorbing capacity of water, which is one of the greatest for any known substance.

You will notice we qualified that last statement by using the phrase "water in its liquid state." This is because, when water changes states from a liquid to a solid or gas, even more extraordinary heat exchanges take place.

For each degree centigrade one gram of water is cooled toward the freezing point, one calorie of heat is given off. However, after that one gram of water has reached 0° C (32° F), approximately 80 calories of heat must be lost before it can change state from liquid to solid. In other words, freezing water gives off 80 times as much heat as an equivalent amount of water being lowered 1° C. These extra calories are known as "latent heat." This means that if you had one gram of water at 80° C, it would require a heat loss of approximately 160 calories to turn it into ice. 80 calories of heat would have to be lost to get the water to 0° C (the freezing point), and then an additional 80 calories of latent heat would have to be lost for it to become ice. The significance of this for hydrotherapy is the following: if freezing water gives off large quantities of latent heat, then melting ice absorbs large quantities of latent heat. One gram of melting ice absorbs 80 times more heat than one gram of water being raised from 0 to 1° C. This makes the ice pack a very powerful treatment.

What happens at the other end of the scale is even more remarkable, and it involves another concept you will remember from chemistry, "heat of vaporization." Heat of vaporization is the energy necessary to evaporate a given mass of liquid. The heat of vaporization of water is 540 calories per gram. This means that while it takes one calorie to heat a gram of water from 99 to 100° C, it takes 540 calories to turn that gram of 100° C water into steam. Likewise, when that gram of steam condenses, it will give off 540 times as much heat as will be given off when it cools from 100 to 99° C. The implication of this for the Russian bath and other hydrotherapeutic measures which employ steam is obvious. As we will point out when we study the Russian bath, the heat from a steam bath does not come primarily from the temperature of the steam, but rather from the large quantities of heat given off as the steam condenses. It should also be noted that water need not be boiled into or condensed from steam for this phenomenon of heat of vaporization to come into play. When evaporation of water takes place at any temperature, the same large quantities of heat are absorbed. This makes the wet sheet pack a powerful treatment.

To recapitulate our first point: water's high specific heat makes it a powerful medium when applied as a liquid; but when it freezes and melts, it is 80 times more powerful; and when it vaporizes and condenses, it is 540 times more powerful. You should also remember that freezing and condensation give off heat and that melting and evaporation absorb heat.

The second of our three important characteristics of water is its fluidity, which makes it easy to apply. If water is the medium for delivering therapeutic heat, then the skin is the medium for the reception of that heat. Through baths and flexible compresses we can "bend" water into just about any shape to conform to the contours of body parts. This allows the effects of its temperature to be mediated through the skin. The nature of these effects is what we will focus on in the next lecture. This ability of water to conform to body shapes is almost as important as its ability to absorb and give off heat.

The third basic property of water we want to mention is its ability to conduct heat. Water carries heat to and away from the body rapidly.

While water is not so efficient a heat conductor as certain metals, it carries heat to and from the body over 25 times faster than air. This is why you can tolerate a 120 ° F sauna but not a 120 ° F hot tub. This is also why it is so dangerous to fall into water during the winter.

To review quickly our introductory points: hydrotherapy is really thermotherapy, and, as such, is a powerful modality which must be used with care and precision.

To review the most basic properties of water: its high specific heat allows it to absorb and give off large quantities of heat; its fluidity allows it to come into easy contact with treatment areas; and its conduction properties allow it to transfer heat effectively.

6. PRINCIPLES OF HOT AND COLD

If hydrotherapy is really thermotherapy, i.e., the treatment of disease by hot and cold, then to learn hydrotherapy we must understand the physiological effects of hot and cold. A lecture on hot and cold should be straightforward. We'll try to keep it that way, but complexities will arise.

Let's begin by defining hot and cold in terms of temperature. For hydrotherapeutic purposes hot is considered to be between 98-104° F, and cold is considered to be between 51-65° F. The following chart defines the full range of temperature possibilities.

TERM	RANGE	COMMENTS
Dangerously hot	125 °F	possibly injurious
Painfully hot	111-124	intolerable
Very hot	105-110	tolerable for short periods
Hot	*98-104*	*tolerable but parts turn red*
Warm or neutral	93-97	comfortable
Tepid	81-92	slightly below skin temperature
Cool	66-80	produces goose flesh
Cold	*55-65*	*tolerable but uncomfortable*
Very cold	32-54	painfully cold

In this chart we have drawn special attention to "hot" and "cold" by italicizing them and putting asterisks by them. For right now these two are the most important concepts to understand.

Having defined hot and cold in terms of temperature, let's now define them in terms of their effects upon the body's circulation. To do this we must define them in terms of duration because their effects change depending on the length of the application.

The circulatory effects of a short hot application are not the same as the effects of a long hot application; in fact, their effects are opposite. A short hot application, defined as one lasting less than five minutes, is stimulating to the circulation. We consider this to be an "intrinsic" effect, meaning it is the direct result of the heat which is transferred to the body. A long hot application, defined as one lasting more than five minutes, is depressing to the circulation. We consider this to be a "reactive" or reflexive effect, meaning it is the result of the body's protective reaction to the heat applied to it.

As we might expect, the circulatory effects of a short cold application are the opposite of the effects of a long cold application, but the scheme for understanding the effects of cold is not identical to the one just outlined for hot. While a short cold application is stimulating to the circulation, it is defined by duration as lasting less than one minute instead of five. And this stimulating effect is considered to be reactive. The effect of a long cold application, i.e., one lasting longer than one minute, is depressing to the circulation and is considered to be an intrinsic or a direct mechanical effect. The following chart lays out these differences in summary form.

APPLICATION	DURATION	EFFECT ON CIRCULATION	CHARACTER
Short hot	< 5 min.	Stimulative	Intrinsic
Long hot	> 5 min.	Depressive	Reactive
Short cold	< 1 min.	Stimulative	Reactive
Long cold	> 1 min.	Depressive	Intrinsic

A close look at the above chart reveals that duration is more predictive of the effects than temperature. Short applications are stimulative regardless of whether they are hot or cold. But how can hot and cold, which are opposites, have similar effects on the body? Because the body reacts to hot and cold at different speeds. The body perceives cold, which is much further away from normal human body temperature than hot, as a greater threat and reacts quickly to it. If the cold is prolonged, the body's reaction is eventually spent and the intrinsic or depressive effect of cold takes over. The body is less threatened by heat and reacts more slowly. Thus the intrinsic or stimulative effect of hot on the circulation is allowed to express itself before the reaction takes place, but if the heat is prolonged, the reactive, depressive effect overrules.

Note: It is easy to become confused about the actual use of these terms "short hot, " "long cold, " etc. When we refer to a "long" application, we are talking about an application which does not significantly change temperature over time, e.g., a bath where the quantity of water is sufficient to not be influenced by the temperature of the body parts immersed in it or the ambient air surrounding it. Therefore, an application which changes temperature over time, e.g., a compress which is more easily influenced by the temperatures of the body parts and air with which it comes in contact, is by definition "short." A 115° F towel applied to the chest and abdomen for ten minutes, even if it is amply covered by wool blankets, will be reduced in temperature to about 95° F in just five minutes. This means it is a short application even if it lasts ten minutes. A cold towel applied similarly at 55 °F may achieve a temperature of 70 °F or more after one minute and of 80 °F or more after ten minutes. Even though it was applied for ten minutes, its practical effect was that of a short cold application.

Let's take our understanding a step further and define specifically what we mean by the stimulative and depressive effects that hot and cold have on circulation. A cold application has an immediate, momentary and insignificant vasoconstrictive effect (intrinsic) followed directly by a vasodilatory effect (reactive) which, if the application is continued long enough, is followed by another vasoconstrictive effect (intrinsic).

Diagrammatically this can be represented as follows:

cold →	vasoconstriction →	vasodilation →	vasoconstriction
	(I)	(R)	(I)
	(intrinsic)	(reactive)	(intrinsic)

A hot application has an immediate vasodilatory effect (intrinsic) followed by a vasostatic effect (reactive).

Diagrammatically:

hot →	vasodilation →	vasostasis
	(I)	(R)

Having looked at the effects of varying lengths of hot and cold applications on circulation, let's look at their effects on the metabolism of the tissues over which they are applied. A short cold application stimulates the metabolism; a long cold application depresses the metabolism. Some of the metabolic and other physiologic effects of short cold are depicted below:

short cold → ↑ ↑ oxygen absorption
↑ ↑ carbon dioxide excretion
↑ nitrogen absorption and excretion
↑ tissue tone
↑ peripheral white blood cell count
↑ peripheral red blood cell count
↓ blood glucose

These effects are the body's reaction to short cold.

A short hot application stimulates the metabolism, as does a long hot application, but neither stimulates it quite so much as a short cold application. While the body has sophisticated means for regulating its temperature, it cannot overcome the biological fact that metabolism is increased by heat, regardless of its duration, so long as it is within a range compatible with life. Therefore, there is no true reactive phase in the metabolic response to a hot application. Some of these metabolic and other physiologic effects of hot are depicted below:

hot → ↑ O_2 absorption
↑ CO_2 excretion
↓ tissue tone
↓ peripheral white blood cell count
↓ peripheral red blood cell count
↑ blood glucose

For future reference, note some of the significant differences between the physiological consequences of cold and hot applications, e.g., their contrasting effects on blood glucose, tissue tone and red and white blood cell counts.

Also for future reference, let's briefly collate the effects we've discussed on the circulation and the metabolism.

APPLICATION	EFFECT ON CIRCULATION	EFFECT ON METABOLISM
short hot	stimulative	stimulative
**long hot*	*depressive*	*stimulative*
short cold	stimulative	stimulative
long cold	depressive	depressive

The italicized and asterisked entry in the above chart is to draw your attention to the potentially dangerous incompatibility between the circulatory and metabolic effects of long hot. Increased metabolism requires a corresponding increase in circulation to support it, i.e., to bring in the necessary nutritional ingredients and carry off the resultant waste products. If circulation is depressed in an area of increased metabolism, serious consequences, such as tissue infarction, can result.

Let's conclude by integrating all the aspects we've discussed about hot and cold into the following depictions (Figure 1):

FIGURE 1

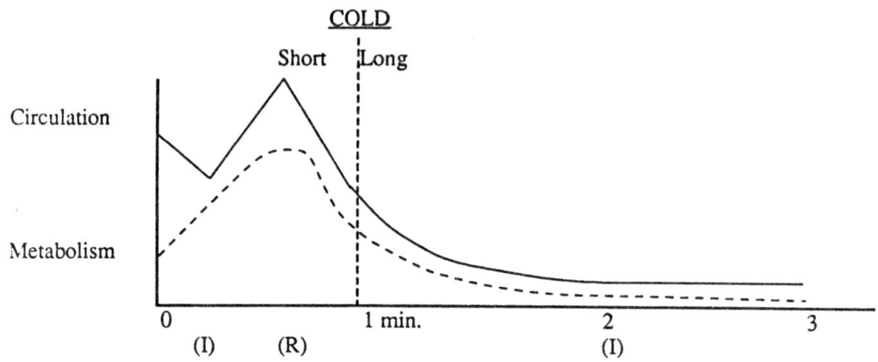

Short cold stimulates and long cold depresses both the circulation and metabolism as reflected by the basically parallel curves in the above graph.

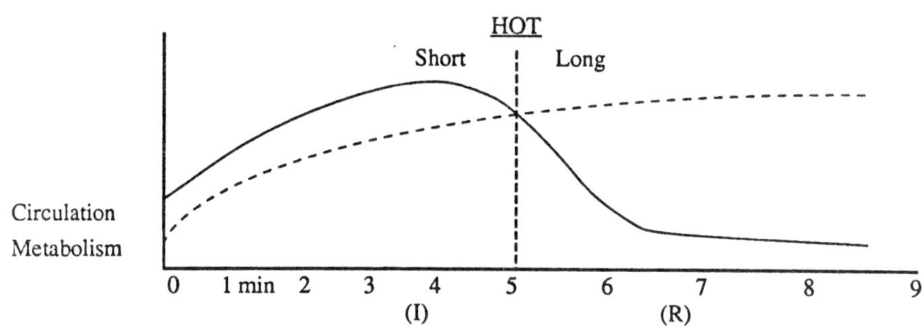

A short hot application stimulates the circulation and metabolism similarly, but if the heat is prolonged, the circulation is depressed to a point which may not be able to adequately support the increased metabolism.

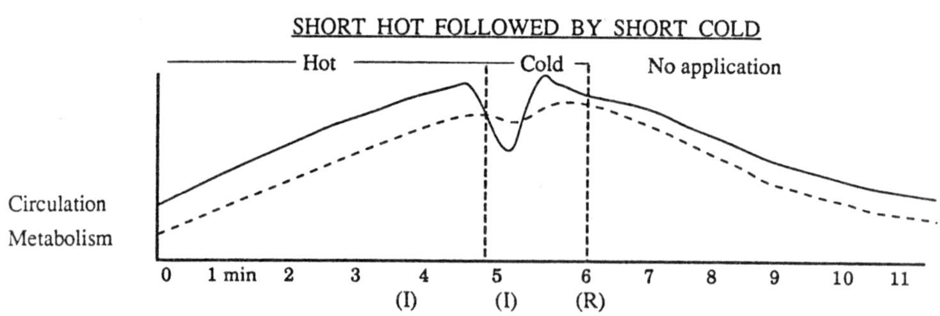

Short hot followed by short cold yields no significant depressive phase for either the circulation or the metabolism. Note the heightened metabolism and circulation is maintained well after such a treatment is terminated.

7. PRINCIPLES OF CIRCULATION

"Pain is the prayer of the nerve for better blood."
— Moritz H. Romberg

If hydrotherapy is based on the premise that healing is proportional to normal blood flow, then as hydrotherapists we must have a good understanding of the circulatory system. This is not the place to go into all the intricacies of circulation, but a brief review of the dynamics of the peripheral circulation, especially of the skin, will serve us well. Remember, the skin is the access organ for hydrotherapy. It is through the skin and the nerves and blood vessels which serve it that the thermal impressions of hydrotherapeutic applications have their impacts upon the body.

The heart gets most of the glory in the circulatory system, and rightly so, for it provides the major force which drives the blood. However, the heart is not the only muscle in the body which pumps blood. You are familiar with the fact that skeletal muscle in the legs and abdomen help pump venous blood back toward the heart. Likewise, the smooth muscle coatings on the arterioles, venules and lymph vessels help move blood along and help maintain the pumping pressure generated by the heart. Even the tiny capillaries, although they do not have a muscular coating, can dilate and constrict and therefore participate in the pumping of blood. In fact, the central heart would be hard put to keep up with the body's circulatory demands without the contractile help of these peripheral vessels. Some writers emphasize the importance of the peripheral vessels to circulation by referring to them collectively as the "peripheral heart" or "skin heart." When you realize that the combined capillary cross-section area is approximately 800 times that of the aorta, you can appreciate that this term is hardly hyperbole. It is a well-known fact that dilated peripheral vessels can act as a reservoir for blood which can almost shut down the central heart by leaving it hardly anything to pump; likewise, abnormally constricted peripheral vessels can overload the central heart.

It is interesting to note that the circulatory principles of dilation and constriction apply to the peripheral heart in much the same way as they do to the central heart. When a peripheral vessel dilates, it fills with blood, and this process is analogous to the diastole in the central heart. When a peripheral vessel contracts, it pushes blood out, and this process is analogous to the systole of the central heart. The dilation and contraction of these peripheral vessels is governed internally by the sympathetic nervous system, oxygen content of the blood, various hormones, etc. As hydrotherapists we are concerned with the mechanical and reflex effects on these processes which can be exerted from the outside by hot and cold — in other words, with how to use hot and cold to cause contraction and/or dilation in the peripheral vessels. We know that the circulatory system is a closed system and that it is therefore impossible to have an effect on one part of the circulation without having effects throughout the system. When a short hot application fills the peripheral vessels and then a short cold application empties and fills them again, significant impact is made on the entire circulatory system, not just the vessels in the skin where the application was made.

Blood makes up approximately 1/13 to 1/12 of the total body weight. Lymph fluid makes up approximately ¼ to ⅓ of the total body weight. This is where hydrotherapy does its work — on the blood and lymph. This is why it can have such a strong impact. Dr. Dick says, "Our job is to nourish and detoxify." These circulating fluids carry nutrients to the vital tissues and carry the toxic by-products away to the organs of elimination. In effecting changes in the blood, we effect changes in all the tissues which it nourishes and cleanses. Here is the essence of hydrotherapy: heat, the therapeutic agent, is put into water, the vehicle, which is applied to the skin (the port-of-entry to the body); the nervous system responds to the thermic impressions and causes changes in the circulation of the blood and lymph which lead to changes at the cellular, tissue, organ and system levels of the body.

We have already talked about the intrinsic or direct versus the reactive or reflexive effects of hot and cold on the body. The reactive or reflexive effects, we noted, are mediated through the nerves. A hot application starts a process which cycles through the spinal cord and results in vasodilation at the site of the application. This parallels the process instigated by a tap over the patellar tendon which results in the familiar knee jerk. The body's reflex reactions to hot and cold applications, as we discussed them, were local, i.e., at the sites of the applications, but these local reflex reactions are not the only ones which take place. Similar reflex reactions occur, usually in the deeper tissue overlain by the application, but they may also take place at a great distance from the application. In the words of Kellogg, "Every portion of the cutaneous surface is in special reflex relation with some internal organ or vascular area." The most important of these are illustrated on the following page in Figure 2.

FIGURE 2
(REFLEX AREAS)

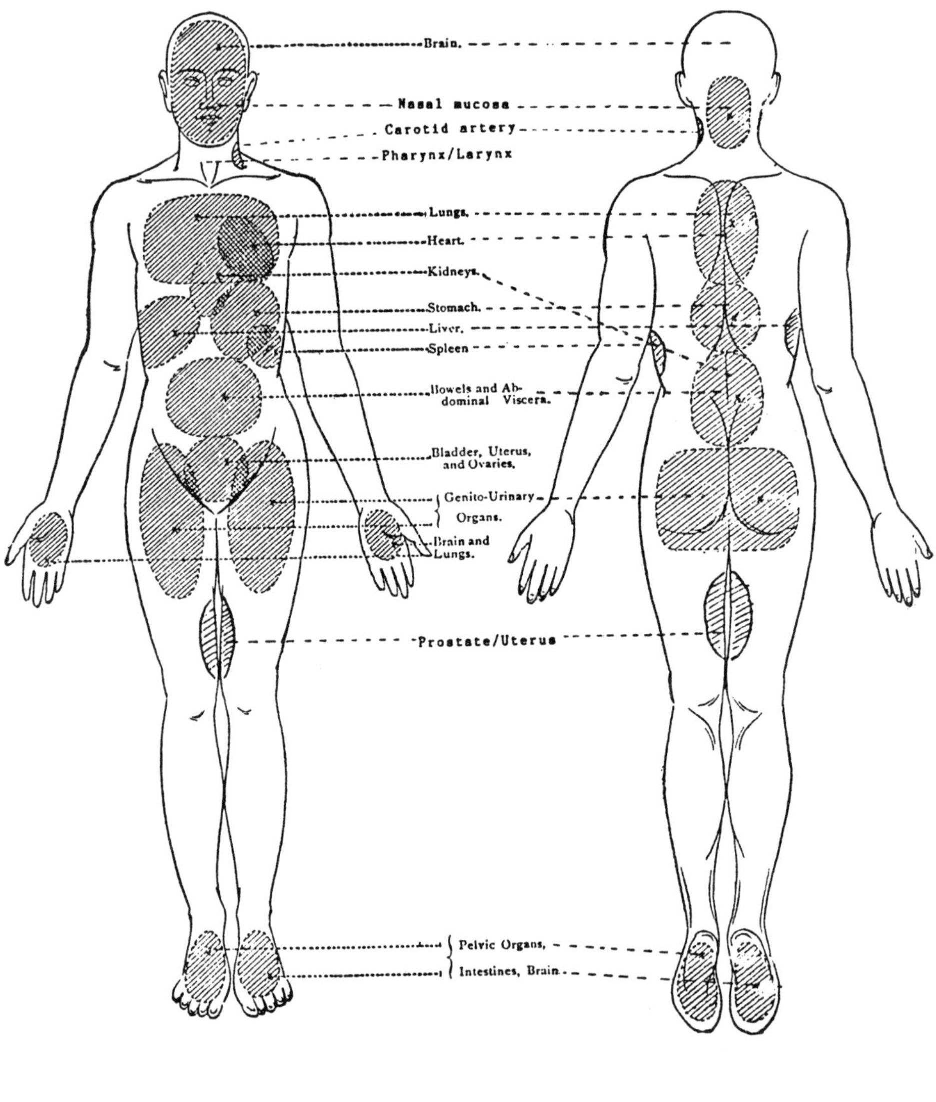

It is important to note that the reflex effects on the deep or distant organs are the same as the direct effects on the skin.

Let's look at the illustration in Figure 2 and run through a couple examples to make sure we understand these reflex areas. Let's take applications to the back of the neck. These would reflexively influence the nasal mucosa. A short hot application to that area would be stimulative (intrinsic) and cause dilation. A long hot application would be depressive (reactive) and cause dilation and stasis. A long cold application would be depressive (intrinsic) and cause vasoconstriction. Which application, then, would you use to stop a bloody nose? The obvious answer is long cold.

What effect would a short cold douche to the sacrum do to uterine vessels? It would cause dilation.

What would a long cold application to the scalp do to the vessels of the brain? It would constrict them.

8. MANIPULATION OF CIRCULATION BY HOT AND COLD

> "The rate of the flow of the blood determines the state of nutrition and the functioning of every cell in the body."
>
> — Frederick Erdman

There are six basic methods hydrotherapists can use to manipulate blood flow. Some of these we have covered, or at least referred to, while others are completely new. For the sake of clarity we will now lay them all out here together.

First is the *direct* method. This involves the local effects about which we have been talking — the effects, both stimulative and depressive which take place in the superficial tissue immediately in contact with the application. These direct effects come unavoidably into play in all applications, and, while they are quite simple, they can be very effective in treating such localized superficial infections as cellulitis of the hand.

Second is the *revulsive or alternate* method. This involves the alternate application of hot and cold. This is really just an elaboration or variation on the direct method which we just discussed. The hot application magnifies the effect of the cold which follows it, which, in turn, increases the effect of the next hot application and so forth. The effects of these applications, when done in alternating sequence, add up to more than they would if they were done separately at widely spaced intervals. This type of application maximizes the peripheral heart and is a very effective decongestant and analgesic. This is one of the most powerful local treatments.

The third method relies on the principles of *derivation and retrostasis.* Derivation is the drawing of blood or lymph from one part of the body by increasing the amount of blood or lymph to another part; retrostasis is the driving of blood or lymph from one area of the body to another area. This method employs the effects of hot and cold on a body-wide basis to move blood and lymph from one area to another. Heat is the mechanism of derivation, which is to say that blood tends to flow toward heat; cold is the mechanism of retrostasis, which is to say that blood tends to flow away from cold. For a person with a congestive headache we can give a derivative treatment consisting of a hot foot bath to the feet. This draws blood and lymph to the feet and away from the head, thus helping to reduce congestion in the painful area. We could also give such a patient a retrostatic treatment consisting of an ice bag to the head. This would drive blood and lymph from the congested head to the lower parts of the body. More effective still would be to combine these complementary treatments, i.e., give hot to the feet and cold to the head. This combination of derivative and retrostatic techniques is one of the safest, cheapest and most reliable treatments you can offer to a patient with a congestive headache.

An important principle of derivation which should be kept in mind is this: in a healthy person with normal circulation a derivative treatment draws blood equally from all other parts; however, in a sick person where there is circulatory congestion, a derivative treatment draws proportionally more blood from the congested parts.

A fourth method for manipulating circulation is based on the principle of *collateral circulation.* This involves the dynamics of derivation and retrostasis which we have just discussed but in a much more restricted area. In derivation and retrostasis circulatory changes in one part of the body are used to affect the circulation in another, distant part. In collateral circulation blood flow modifications in a superficial artery are used to change the circulation of a deep artery from the same trunk. To understand this better please consult Figure 3 on the following page.

FIGURE 3

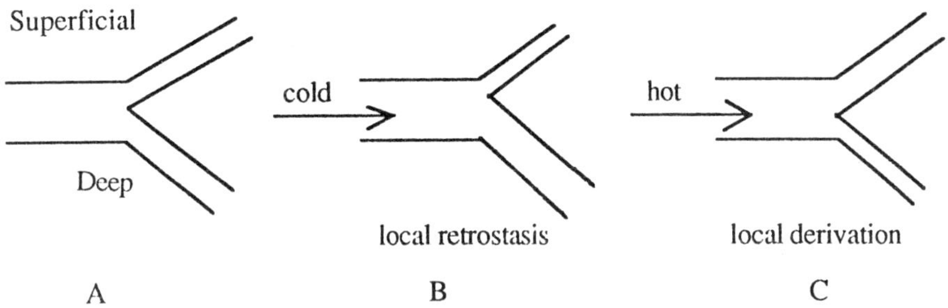

When an arterial trunk bifurcates into superficial and deep branches, and the circulation is normal, blood flow through the two branches is roughly equal. This is represented by diagram A in Figure 3. If cold were applied over the start of the superficial branch, that branch would constrict, and blood flow through it would decrease, while, at the same time, the deep branch would dilate and blood flow through it would increase. This would represent a retrostatic reaction. See diagram B in Figure 3. If hot were applied to the superficial branch, the results would be the opposite, i.e., the superficial vessel would dilate and pass more blood, while the deep branch would constrict and pass less blood. This would be a local derivative reaction. See diagram C in Figure 3.

An example of such an application would be in the arm where the radial and ulnar arteries split off from the brachial. The radial artery is superficial and the ulnar artery is deep. We can influence the radial artery directly and the ulnar artery indirectly by making the kinds of applications described above.

The *arterial trunk reflex* represents a fifth way to manipulate circulation. This is based on the principle that whatever influence is exerted on an arterial trunk will be conveyed to the smaller vessels fed by that trunk. If we apply hot to an arterial trunk, we find that not only does the arterial trunk dilate and carry more blood but so do the distal arteries branching off from the trunk. This is an important principle to be acquainted with in hydrotherapeutic management of such conditions as diabetic leg ulcers where hot applications to the extremities are contraindicated. A small hot application over the femoral artery will cause dilation in the anterior tibial artery, thus increasing circulation in the compromised area without dangerously raising the local metabolic rate.

If we apply cold to an arterial trunk, we find constriction of the trunk as well as of the distal vessels fed by it. Therefore, in case of hemorrhage following a cut on the foot, an ice pack over the femoral artery would cause constriction in the dorsalis pedis artery and help control bleeding. This is much like using pressure over an arterial trunk to stop bleeding; in fact, cold and pressure may be combined over an arterial trunk for an even stronger hemostatic effect.

The sixth method for controlling circulation involves the *spinal cord reflex*. We went into this in some detail in the previous lesson. It is based on the principle that each vital center has a corresponding area of skin which is reflexively connected to it. For example, a long cold application to the skin over the spleen would result in constriction of the skin vessels overlying the spleen as well as constriction of the splenic vessels. A short hot application over the liver would result in dilation of the skin vessels overlying the liver as well as dilation of the hepatic vessels.

An important extension of this principle applies to the symmetrically paired structures of the body. For example, the left hand is reflexively related through the spinal cord to the right hand and vice versa, just as the right shoulder is reflexively related through the cord to the left shoulder. What is the clinical significance of this? If you want to speed healing to a fractured left foot which is not accessible to hydrotherapeutic applications because it is in a cast, you may make alternate hot and cold applications to the healthy, accessible right foot. Please take note of this little trick, as situations like this arise with surprising frequency.

Now, any intelligent student will see that certain hydrotherapeutic treatments can yield conflicting results according to the principles we have just stated. For example, a hot foot bath will draw blood away from the head via derivation yet increase blood flow to the head via the spinal cord reflex. In such a case, how do you know which principle predominates? Here are some guidelines to help you judge:

1) the smaller the area of the application, the more the effects tend to be reflexive, e.g., the strongest effect of an ice bag to the inside of the thighs will be constriction of the uterine or prostate vessels;

2) the larger the area of the application, the more the effects tend to be direct, e.g., a hot full-body bath does not have so great a total effect on the reflex points it covers as would occur if the reflex points were stimulated individually;

3) the greater the intensity of the application,the more the effects tend to be reflexive, e.g., a very cold application to the hand would give strong local and reflexive effects (to the brain) but a neutral application (e.g., 93 ° C) would have primarily local effects;

4) the closer the area of application is to the reflex organ, the more the effects tend to be reflexive, e.g., an application over the head or heart tends to be strongly reflexive in its effects on the respective underlying organ; whereas the further away the area of application is from the reflex organ, the more the effects tend to be direct or mechanical, e.g., a hot foot bath tends to have a stronger derivative than reflex effect because of the great distance between the feet and the brain, lungs and bladder to which they are reflexively related.

Of course these variables can interact and modify any application, e.g., a very small, very hot applicaton to the foot would generate stronger reflexive reactions than a standard hot foot bath.

To conclude, let's apply all six basic principles for manipulating circulation by hot and cold to a single case.

For cerebral congestion we could apply:

1) (direct) cold to the head
2) (revulsive) alternate hot and cold to the head
3) (derivative/retrostatic) cold to the head and hot to the feet
4) (collateral) hot to the face over the maxillary artery (thus drawing blood away from the middle meningeal artery which branches deep to the brain)

5) (arterial trunk) ice pack to the carotids
6) (spinal cord reflex) cold to the palms

9. PRINCIPLES OF HYDROTHERAPY

The following principles of hydrotherapy are mostly an integration and clarification of previous material but with a few new ideas added in. We think it is important to address the basic principles of hydrotherapy from several directions so that they may be thoroughly recognized and understood.

We mentioned in our introduction to this course that it is the hydrotherapist's job to manipulate the clinical variables under his or her control in a fashion appropriate to the clinical variables outside his or her control such as the patient's condition, vitality, etc. We will first run through six important treatment variables under the hydrotherapist's control which should be taken into account in formulating effective hydrotherapies.

The first variable is the *temperature* of the application. The greater the difference between the temperature of the application and the body temperature, the greater the intensity of the treatment. For example, a five-minute sitz bath at 55 ° F is a stronger treatment than a five-minute sitz bath at 70 ° F, just as a five-minute sitz bath at 105 ° F is a stronger treatment than one at 100 ° F. In alternate or revulsive treatments the greater the contrast in temperature between the hot and cold applications, the greater the intensity of the treatment. Therefore, a hot foot bath at 105 ° F followed by a cold foot bath of 40 ° F is a stronger treatment than a hot foot bath of 100 ° F followed by a cold foot bath at 55 ° F.

The second important variable is *timing,* and under timing are several sub-categories. First is *duration* of the application. When the temperature of the application is extreme, the duration is inversely proportional to the overall intensity of the treatment. This reflects what we discussed early in the course — that a short hot or cold treatment is stimulative to the circulation, while a long hot or cold treatment is depressive. For example, a one-minute sitz bath at 50° F is a more stimulating treatment than a ten-minute sitz bath at 50° F. Likewise, a five-minute full-body bath at 111° F would be a stronger treatment than a twenty-minute full-body bath at the same temperature. However, at moderate temperatures the intensity of the treatment is directly proportional to the duration of that treatment. A two-hour neutral bath at 94° F is a stronger treatment than a half-hour bath at the same temperature.

The next sub-category under timing is *frequency.* The more frequently an application is made, the more intense the overall effect. In a strong patient the effectiveness of the repeated treatment is enhanced, but in a weak patient the increased intensity of the repeated treatments reduces their effectiveness. Keep in mind that the first treatment is the most intense. The strength of each repetition is reduced until a point of diminishing returns is reached as the body's reactive capacities are exhausted.

Also under timing we include the *hour of the day* the treatment is given. If you give the hydrotherapy at the patient's strong time of the day, the effectiveness is enhanced. If you give the treatment at the patient's weak time of the day, the effectiveness is diminished. The patient's best and worst times of the day are as important for the hydrotherapist as for the homeopath. We talk about individualizing treatments, and the time the therapy is given is an important and neglected aspect of this.

The third treatment variable is the *location* or *site* of the application. Obviously, the *reflex areas* we have already discussed are important here (see page 38). Along with the location, another important consideration is the *extent* of the application. In derivative measures, the greater the treatment area, the greater the intensity of the treatment. For congestive headache a hot full-body bath is a stronger derivative treatment than a hot foot bath, because a greater volume of blood and lymph can be pulled into the larger treatment region. In retrostatic measures, the opposite holds. The smaller the treatment area, the more intense the effect. For a sprained ankle a cold foot bath has a stronger retrostatic effect than a cold leg and foot bath, because the smaller the bath, the more area there is to push the congested fluids to. Extent of the application also comes into play in alternate and revulsive treatments. As we will discuss later, the cold application in these cases should be smaller than the preceding hot application. It is also important to know that the greater the size difference between the hot and cold applications, the greater the intensity of their combined effect. For example, a hot trunk compress followed by a cold umbilical compress is a stronger treatment than a hot trunk compress followed by a cold abdominal compress.

The fourth variable involves the application of either *pressure* or *friction.* A pressure application would usually take the form either of an external douche or an affusion. The greater force with which the water hits the body, the greater the intensity of the treatment. For example, a douche in the form of a stream of 105 ° F water sprayed under 20 pounds of pressure against the calf is a stronger treatment than such a douche at 10 pounds pressure, which, in turn, would be stronger than a 105 ° F leg bath. Likewise, a one-gallon affusion of 60 ° F water to the back poured from six feet is a stronger treatment than one poured from two feet. Not only does the pressure increase the intensity of the treatment, it also increases the patient's ability to tolerate extreme temperatures, probably via the gate-theory mechanism. Therefore, a patient can more comfortably tolerate a 60 ° F pressure shower than a 60 ° F bath. All these things hold true for friction as well. A 45 ° F ablution applied with strong friction with a coarse friction mitt is a much stronger treatment than a 45 ° F ablution given lightly with a smooth hand. Likewise, the ablution with heavy friction would feel warmer than the ablution with weak friction. The pressure and friction not only send nervous stimuli which compete with and diminish the perception of cold, but also bring blood to the surface which warms the cutaneous tissue and helps quiet the cold receptors.

A fifth treatment variable which applies specifically to compresses concerns the *material* used for covering the compress. The ability of water vapor to penetrate the covering is inversely proportional to the heating effects of the compress. That is to say, that a heating compress covered by plastic and wool will cut down on cooling through evaporation and promote a stronger heating, and therefore derivative, response. A heating compress covered only by wool will lose water vapor and heat more readily and result in a more tonic reaction.

The sixth variable, which again is specifically applicable to compresses and fomentations, has to do with the *wetness* of the application. The wetter the application, the stronger the temperature impact on the body. A towel loosely wrung out in 115° F water carries more heat than a towel tightly wrung out in 115° F water. When we get to the constitutional treatment, you will see that we grade how tightly we wring out the cold towels according to the vitality of the patient. On a chilly, debilitated rheumatic patient we reduce the impact of the cold compress by wringing it to a relatively dry state.

So the temperature, timing, location, pressure, covering and wetness of your applications are the variables under your control. You must learn to use your own clinical judgement on how to manipulate these variables to create a hydrotherapy appropriate to the individual patient and his or her peculiar clinical needs.

Beyond these controlled variables are other important principles of hydrotherapy. Again, many of these have already been mentioned, but to emphasize these vital rules, we would like to list them together as the *15 Commandments of Hydrotherapy.*

15 Commandments of Hydrotherapy.

1. Always explain the hydrotherapeutic procedures ahead of time to the patient. This includes the length, sequence, frequency, cost, rationale, cold, etc. Don't surprise your patients.
2. Always take the patient's body temperature before each treatment and adjust your treatment accordingly, e.g., if a patient's temperature were below normal, you might want to intensify the hot portion of the treatment and decrease the intensity of the

cold portion. It is also a good idea to take the patient's temperature after each treatment to help gauge treatment response.

3. In a prolonged hot treatment, always monitor the patient's pulse and temperature. In a strong patient the pulse should be kept below 140 beats per minute and the temperature below 104° F. In a weaker patient the allowable limits would be even less.
4. Treat the young, old, obese, and feeble with care, especially in terms of cold applications, because of their poor capacity to respond to intense treatments. This is another way of saying: know well all the contraindications of your treatments.
5. Make precise prescriptions for your treatments. This is of utmost importance if you are not performing the treatments yourself. Even if you are your own technician, it is still important to have a clear, written record of prescribed hydrotherapy treatments, not only for legal reasons, but also for research and learning purposes, and so that treatments which are not producing desired results can be intelligently adjusted, and ones which are producing good results can be repeated consistently.
6. If the patient is chilled by the treatment, i.e., if he or she feels chilly or shows goose flesh, stop the treatment immediately and warm the patient by applying heat, friction, blankets, giving warm drinks, etc.
7. Treat the patient before — not after — meals.
8. Treat the patient at his or her "strong" but not "weak" time of the day.
9. Always allow time and space for a rest period after each treatment.
10. Avoid excess heat after treatment.
11. In a prolonged series of treatments, monitor patient medications and watch for signs of healing crisis (see Chapter 32).
12. Always precede cold with hot. There are possible exceptions to this, but this is the general rule.
13. Always make the hot application bigger and longer than the cold application. Note the following diagram (Figure 4).

FIGURE 4

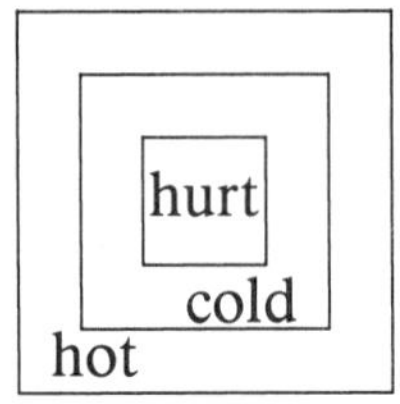

14. *Always end with cold**.*
15. *Always cover compresses with wool.***

Please remember these last two commandments. If we failed to inculcate these into you, Dr. Dick would never forgive us.

10. FEVER AND NATUROPATHIC HYDROTHERAPY

Treatment of febrile cases will come up when we discuss management of acute disease, but we would like to devote a whole lecture to the subject here, as it is central to our understanding of naturopathic hydrotherapy.

Fever may be defined as an increase in regulated body temperature resulting from an elevation in the thermoregulatory "set point." It is distinct from elevations of body temperature (hyperthermia) due to exercise, passive heating (steam baths, saunas, sunbathing, etc.) or a breakdown in the ability to regulate body temperature (heat stroke or malignant hyperthermia.) As hydrotherapists we are primarily concerned with increases in regulated body temperature resulting from infectious disease.

We've talked before about the secret of hydrotherapy. What is the secret meaning of fever? In infectious disease, fever is the body treating itself with thermotherapy.

How does the body create fever in infectious disease? A microbial product from the infecting organism known as the *exogenous pyrogen* is phagocytized by a macrophage. This results in the release of interleukin-1, also known as ***endogenous pyrogen***. This endogenous pyrogen, or fever producer, travels hormone-like via the blood to the hypothalamus and stimulates the production of prostaglandin E_2 (PGE_2) which causes the body temperature set-point or thermostat to be turned up. The body now perceives its normal temperature as too low and begins to generate more heat by shivering and by putting into circulation more thyrotropin-releasing factor while conserving heat by vasoconstriction, which limits blood flow to the cooling surfaces of the body, and by piloerection, which shuts down the sweating mechanism. These heat-conservative measures are mediated through the sympathetic nervous system and are perceived as chills. In the hypothalamus interleukin-1 will also provoke sleep to help the host preserve energy for internal defense. In the liver it promotes the production of special proteins (C-reactive protein, ceruloplasmin, complement system components, haptoglobulins, fibrinogen, etc.) to aid immunity and increase protection against hepatocellular damage from endotoxins. While all this is happening, interleukin-1 also goes via the blood to skeletal muscle and stimulates the release of PGE_2 in that tissue. This promotes lysosomal activity which leads to a breakdown in muscle tissue. The postural muscles are the most susceptible to this. This is why aches in the back and legs are common with fever and chills. The increase in the body's amino acid pool resulting from the muscle protein breakdown provides the body with raw materials for defense, repair and energy as well as depressing the appetite. When you add to this the ability of interleukin-1 to produce anorexia by decreasing gut motility you can understand why a feverish child who has not had his appetite perverted will not eat while he is sick.

Why does the body go through all these various and intricate changes? Because they have survival value. Because it is an effective defense mechanism. It is, in fact, the *Vis Medicatrix Naturae* at work.

When the body temperature is elevated in fever, white blood cell production is increased as is the rate of white blood cell release into the circulation. At the same time, white blood cell mobility and killing ability is enhanced, the production of interferon is speeded up and antibody production is increased up to 20 times. What is the meaning of this? Fever is an immune system stimulant.

While fever is cranking up the body's defenses, it is also providing an inhospitable environment for the invading organism. As body temperature rises, blood concentrations of iron and zinc are reduced, which inhibits bacterial growth. At a temperature of 104 ° F gonococcus is killed, and the polio virus growth rate is reduced by 250 times. At 106 ° F pneumococcus dies, as do spirochetes. You may be aware that the discovery that there was no tertiary syphilis in malarial areas led to the routine infection of syphilitics with malaria as standard treatment before antibiotics became available. Between 106-110° F malignant cells are selectively destroyed. Some cancer clinics are employing various hyperthermia techniques to fight cancer. At temperatures greater than 110° F normal cells die, depending on the length of exposure.

This accounts for the benefits of increased temperature, but what about the breakdown of muscle tissue and the build-up of the amino acid pool? As already mentioned, the increase in the amino acid pool depresses the appetite. This is important because the digestive system shuts down when body temperature (oral) goes above 99.5° F. If food is taken during fever, it will strain the system and, by not being properly digested, will add to the toxic load of the body, inhibiting its ability to deal with the cause of the fever. Therefore, this appetite suppression is a protective mechanism which allows the body's energies to be concentrated on the problem causing the fever. At the same time this increased amino acid pool provides the raw materials needed for rapid antibody synthesis to help in fighting off the invading organisms without the damaging intake of food. The simple elegance of this protective mechanism is typical of the *Vis Medicatrix Naturae.*

Some interesting animal experiments by Kluger and others shed light on the value of fever in infectious disease. Coldblooded animals (lizards) were artificially infected and placed in cages where the temperature was graded, with the coolest temperature at the bottom of the cage and the warmest temperature at the top. All the infected lizards gravitated to the upper parts of the cage toward the higher temperature. A similar experiment was done with fish, all of which sought warmer water after being infected. This was taken a step further by restricting the movement of some of the infected fish. There was a 100% recovery rate among the infected fish which were free to migrate to the warmer water. There was a 0% recovery rate among the fish which were prevented from swimming to the warmer water. In another experiment rabbits were inoculated with pneumococcus and divided into two groups. The first group was untreated and had a death rate of 29%. The second group had their fevers reduced by 1° C or 1.5° F with salicylates. The death rate among this fever-suppressed group was 100%.

Hippocrates, the Father of Medicine, said, "Give me a fever, and I can cure any disease," because he knew that fever signaled the arousal of the body's defenses to fight off disease. He felt that the higher the fever, the better his results would be. William Osler, the supposed Father of Modern Medicine, said "Fever, famine and war are the great enemies of humanity, and the greatest and most terrible is fever." As naturopathic physicians, we proudly subscribe to the Hippocratic rather than the Oslerian tradition. We are not afraid of fever but regard it as our ally. This does not mean that we do not recognize potential dangers in fever. We regard 98.6° F as normal temperature, 102-103° F as optimal for fighting infectious disease, 104-107° F as the point where dehydration becomes a serious concern, and fevers above 107° F as frankly dangerous.

Most harm associated with high fevers is usually due to dehydration, electrolyte imbalance or the cause of the fever rather than the fever itself. Extensive search in the literature has failed to reveal a single case of brain damage due to temperature elevation caused by infection except in meningitis and encephalitis which may themselves cause brain damage. We must remember that patients undergoing hyperthermia are maintained at temperatures of 108° F (42.2° C) for 10-12 hours.

In a properly managed case, fever will not go to these dangerous levels. Dr. Herbert Shelton says that if you fast a fever patient, the temperature will never go too high. Clinical experience shows that a fever will rarely go above 104° F in an adult if you do not feed the patient. In infants and young children fever may occasionally reach 105° F for a short time even when properly managed. Remember what we said about the digestive system shutting down above 99.5° F. If you feed a feverish patient, you are interfering with his body's attempt to overcome the disease and are in danger of running the fever to harmful levels.

It goes without saying that you do not suppress fever with antipyretic drugs such as aspirin. This has always been a firm naturopathic principal, and now even orthodox medicine recognizes its validity because of the link between aspirin administration and Reye's syndrome in flu and chicken pox, etc. Acetaminophen is no better and totally unnecessary. If a fever must absolutely be brought down, a tepid friction rub is the treatment of choice.

The higher the fever, the better it is – André Saine

What about febrile seizures? This is the big bugaboo with fever in children. First, remember that most febrile seizures are the result of imbalanced electrolytes due to dehydration from diarrhea, vomiting and increased perspiration and respiration. Second, remember that anticonvulsant drugs do not prevent the development of epilepsy in patients with febrile seizures and should therefore not be administered on that basis. They should be allowed only in cases where there are EEG abnormalities or where the seizure has lasted longer than 15 minutes. Keep in mind our homeopathic remedies such as *Belladonna, Hyoscyamus, Nux vomica* and *Strammonium* which can affect convulsions with heat and may help to abort a febrile seizure if the overall symptom picture matches. Such hydrotherapeutic measures as cold to the spine and hot to the head, followed by hot to the spine and cold to the head may also be helpful. In any case, do not allow a seizure to go beyond 15 minutes. Febrile seizures lasting substantially longer can lead to brain damage from hypoxia due to airway blockage or from constant seizing but not due to the elevated temperature itself. However, good management in the form of limiting food and maintaining fluids and electrolytes will prevent most cases from progressing to the more critical stages. As naturopathic hydrotherapists we seek to maximize the good effects of fever and minimize the potential dangers during fever.

If fever is the body treating itself with thermotherapy, and if hydrotherapy is treating the body with thermotherapy, what are the principles governing the hydrotherapeutic management of the febrile patient? The first goal of hydrotherapy in febrile illness is to help the body maintain its temperature at the optimal level (while individually variable, about 102-103 °F on average) for fighting infection. This means lowering dangerously high fever or even intensifying a low fever. Other goals of hydrotherapy are to boost immunity and improve the circulation which we have already discussed. Of course, you rest febrile patients and fast them unless otherwise indicated, as, for example, in diabetics, and you keep them well hydrated with special attention to electrolytes, expecially if diarrhea or vomiting is present.

Let's go into more detail about how to use water to control a high fever in cases when it may become necessary. In this, our attention will be focused on the skin. It is the route of entry for the thermic impressions of hydrotherapy, it is the primary route for the elimination of heat (about 75%), and it is reflexively related to organs and muscles which produce body heat.

There are two important aspects of fever to consider — heat production and heat elimination. Let's look at the effects various hydrotherapeutic applications of different durations and temperatures have on these two factors, all else being equal. A short cold application increases the heat loss and the heat production for basically no net change in the body temperature, while a long cold treatment would lead to a heat loss combined with a decrease in heat production for a modest net loss of body temperature. The heat loss here is not so great as one might expect due to the fact that the long cold application drives the heat-carrying blood to the inner reservoirs. A tepid application actually results in a larger net heat loss. Even though it causes no change in heat production,the elimination of heat is effective because the circulation to the periphery is relatively undisturbed. A long hot application would result in decreased heat elimination and increased production for a net increase in body temperature. A short hot treatment of 3-5 minutes would also reduce heat elimination and increase heat production, but a very short hot application of less than a minute would increase heat elimination because of vasodilation and perspiration and would result in only an insignificant rise in heat production for a modest net loss of body heat. The following chart (Figure 5) summarizes this.

FIGURE 5

DURATION/TEMP.	HEAT ELIMINATION	HEAT PRODUCTION	NET CHANGE
short cold	↑	↑	no change
long cold	↑	↓ unless shivering results	↓
tepid	↑	no change	↓
long hot	↓	↑	↑
short hot	↓	↑	↑
very short hot	↑	↑	↓

The only applications offering a net loss in body heat are the long cold, tepid and very short hot, and none of these are dramatic in their effect. Some other factor must come into play, and that factor is *friction*. Not only does friction allow the patient to tolerate a cold treatment better, but it draws the heat-carrying blood to the skin for increased heat elimination. At the same time, blood flow to the muscles and organs is reduced which slows down heat production, and the nerves are "warmed," thus cutting down on the reflex production of heat via shivering. Remember, long cold will not be effective in reducing body temperature without friction. Heat is not in the skin; it is in the blood. Cold tends to drive the blood and, therefore, the heat it is trying to capture out of the skin. Then, how do you get the blood to stay at the surface in the presence of cold? *Friction.* Friction is the bait which draws blood to the surface to be cooled. By itself cold reduces blood flow to the skin, reduces heat loss through perspiration and decreases skin conduction of heat. Without friction cold is an enemy in fever reduction.In all fever-reducing treatments you stop the treatment when the febrile patient begins to shiver — not because you do not want them to feel cold, but because shivering will increase heat production, decrease heat elimination and, therefore, raise the temperature you are trying to reduce.

Let's outline some useful antipyretic water applications.

The *tepid affusion* (81-92° F) or the *neutral affusion* (93-96° F) consists of seating the patient in a large tub, such as a regular bath tub, and pouring water at the appropriate temperature over the back of the neck and shoulders until the desired body temperature is reached. (*Please note:* one of the most important principles in all these fever-reducing treatments is not to overshoot your goal as far as the temperature is concerned. You must allow for what we will call the "coasting factor." Oral temperature is not instantaneously responsive to whole-body temperature changes. There is a brief lag time which must be taken into account. If you want to lower the temperature to 102° F, and continue your treatment until the oral temperature reads 102° F, the momentum may carry the temperature down to 100° F. Let's say your patient has a temperature of 106° F and you want to reduce it to 102° F.

You should monitor the oral temperature closely and end the treatment when the temperature reaches around 103.5 ° F and let it coast the rest of the way.) The tepid and/or neutral affusions work by increasing heat elimination through simple conduction without changing heat production. Because these affusions do not inhibit circulation, heat from the blood is readily available to be carried off by the cooler water. The pressure from the poured water enhances this effect.

The *tepid bath* or the *neutral bath* would be at the same temperature as the above affusions, the patient in this case being immersed full-body in a tub of water at the appropriate temperature. The mechanism would be identical; however, there would be no pressure enhancement. In a normal person these baths result in no appreciable change in body temperature, but in fever cases the body temperature is reduced. This is because there is a greater relative difference in the temperatures of the baths and the fever patient, and because the elevated temperatures of fever patients are more susceptible to change.

The *graduated bath* is good to use in fever patients who are weak or intolerant to cooler temperatures. This is a full-body bath begun at 4 ° F below the body temperature. For example, if the patient's temperature is 105 ° F, the graduated bath would be started at 101 ° F. Cooler water is then gradually added to the bath so that the bath temperature is lowered at a rate of approximately 1 ° F every three minutes to 86 ° F or less or until the patient becomes chilly. Gentle friction is also applied. For those extremely intolerant to cold,the treatment may be started at an even hotter temperature. The basic mechanism is the same as the previous baths with the addition of friction to facilitate the cooling effects.

The *Brand bath* was developed by a European army doctor for treating soldiers suffering from typhoid. It is a "heroic" treatment reserved for extreme cases. Questions about the Brand bath have been known to appear on various state board exams. The Brand bath is a cold friction bath, although the temperatures have been moderated somewhat over time. Do not confuse this with the "bran" bath which employs wheat bran in the treatment of certain dermatological disorders. The Brand bath is a whole-body tub immersion (except for the head) at between 70-80 ° F. Whole-body friction is applied vigorously to the entire body except the abdomen. Two people are necessary to do this most effectively. Every few minutes a cold water affusion is given over the head, a towel having previously been wrapped about the head to prevent the cold water from pouring over the face. If the patient becomes chilly, continue the treatment. However, if the patient's teeth start to chatter or if the patient begins to shiver, terminate the treatment. Why? Because the shivering will start to drive the temperature back up. Otherwise,continue the treatment for 10-20 minutes. Monitor oral temperature throughout. If at the end of the treatment it is greater than 103° F, don't dry the patient. If the temperature is less than 103° F, dry the patient. Then wrap the patient in a dry flannel sheet and wool blankets as necessary. Let the patient rest. Take the temperature every half hour.If the temperature increases slowly while in the dry wrap, apply cool compresses to the head. If the temperature increases rapidly, repeat the treatment. If the temperature goes back above 105° F, repeat the treatment. The Brand bath is indicated for high fever, i.e., 105° F or above, when lassitude, restlessness, delirium and/or shallow breathing are present. It is an emergency measure to save patients from a fever which has gone, for whatever reasons, out of control. One treatment may reduce the temperature by as much at 3-4° F, so monitor the oral temperature and remember to allow for the coasting factor. This is a long cold treatment which depresses heat production and increases heat elimination. The friction enhances both these effects as does the pressure from the affusion.

The *hot evaporating sheet* is a good fever treatment to know. In this case you wrap the patient in a sheet wrung out in water as hot as possible. Then apply friction through the sheet and allow the sheet to cool. Manual or electrical fanning may be desirable. Repeat the hot sheet application every five to eight minutes or as the patient becomes chilly. The hot sheet pack is effective because it brings blood to the surface of the skin for more efficient cooling without significantly changing the body's heat production. As water evaporates from the sheet, cooling is accelerated and is further enhanced by fanning. Of course, the friction increases the efficiency of all these.

The *tepid sponge bath* is self-descriptive. Water between 81-92° F is applied to the trunk and arms with a sponge. This is a gentle and effective treatment for fever reduction well suited for use on children. Cooling is by conduction and evaporation. Heat production remains unaffected. The sponging provides a gentle friction which enhances peripheral circulation and, hence, heat loss.

Also, don't forget water drinking. It keeps the febrile patient hydrated, absorbs heat, facilitates toxin elimination through the skin, kidney and bowel, and promotes cooling by evaporation through the skin. Have patient drink to thirst unless otherwise indicated.

Note: If perspiration is present, do not lower the fever with external water applications. Sweating is the body's own mechanism for lowering its temperature, so don't interfere with it. It is doing its job. However, if sweat is absent during high fever, supply the cooling moisture which nature has failed to provide.

Let's conclude this long discussion with the important principles of hydrotherapeutic fever management:

1) Fever is beneficial; don't be afraid of it;
2) Leave fever alone unless it is threatening to go to dangerous levels;
3) Fast the febrile patient, and slowly resume feeding only when the patient recovers natural hunger and his temperature is back below 99.5° F;
4) Leave the sweating patient alone so far as the fever is concerned; don't help the body when it doesn't need it;
5) Remember 102-103° F is considered optimal for infection fighting;
6) Allow for the "coasting factor", i.e., stop treatment before temperature reaches desired level so that you don't overshoot it;
7) Make sure cold treatments are "long," i.e., 10-30 minutes;
8) Always use friction with cold;
9) Always stop the treatment if shivering occurs;
10) Neutral treatments should last from one to three hours.

II.
DEMONSTRATIONS

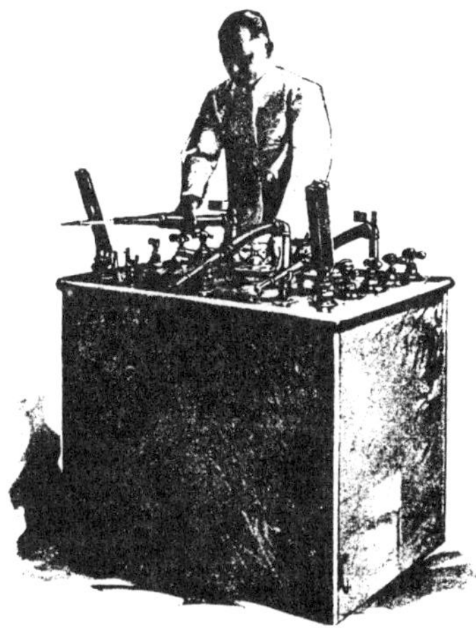

II. INTRODUCTION — HYDROTHERAPY EQUIPMENT AND TEMPERATURE CONVERSIONS

> "In the modern development of hydrotherapy an imposing array of apparatus was devised . . . In proportion as the complexity of the outfits increased their employment in general decreased . . . It is a fact, however, that in trained hands, with no more expensive and complicated implements than a supply of hot and cold water, a bathtub, a few towels and sheets, a multiplicity of remedial effects can be accomplished."
>
> — Richard Kovacs

HYDROTHERAPY EQUIPMENT

Before moving on to our first demonstrations, a few words about the basic materials needed for hydrotherapy are in order.

If there are currently stores specializing in the sale of hydrotherapy equipment other than whirlpools and hot tubs, we are unaware of them. Fortunately, most of the equipment needed for basic hydrotherapy is simple enough that it can be procured from hardwares, department stores and other traditional suppliers of household goods.

Towels are indispensible to hydrotherapy and should be made from white all-cotton terrycloth as should washcloths and friction mitts.

Sheets and compress material should be white and all-cotton or linen. Ideally blankets, fomentations and compress covers should be 100% wool. When outfitting your office we recommend you buy all-natural-fiber materials, but do not get hung up on this issue in terms of home treatments or emergency situations. In some instances, the best equipment is that which is readily at hand. Use your common sense here.

Tubs of appropriate sizes in which to immerse various body parts are necessary. Plastic dishpans make fine foot tubs. Laundry rinse tubs, either plastic or galvanized, make good sitz baths. If you are lucky and diligent, you may even find a "real" sitz tub, such as that pictured on this book's cover, in some out-of-the-way location.

Accurate thermometers for measuring water temperature are essential. Centigrade or Fahrenheit makes no difference so long as the range of temperature calibration is adequate for your purposes. Bath thermometers which are protected from easy breakage are best. Medical and laboratory suppliers carry a variety of these, although you can substitute a regular outdoor thermometer in an emergency. Oral thermometers are frequently required to monitor the patient's body temperature during treatments as well.

Of course, other pieces of equipment are necessary for a full range of hydrotherapy, and these will be discussed later. Those mentioned above are the most basic.

TEMPERATURE CONVERSIONS

The serious hydrotherapist should be able to make quick conversions back and forth between the Centigrade and Fahrenheit temperature scales. The following chart is useful to consult.

Centigrade	Fahrenheit
0	32
5	41
10	50
15	59
20	68
25	77
30	86
35	95
36	96.8
37	98.6
38	100.4
39	102.2
40	104
41	105.8
42	107.6
43	109.4
44	111.2
45	113
50	122
55	131
60	140
65	149
70	158
75	167
80	176
85	185
90	194
95	203
100	212

The formulas for calculating these conversions are as follows:

From Centigrade to Fahrenheit:

$9/5X + 32$ (where X = ° C)

From Fahrenheit to Centigrade:

$\frac{5(X-32)}{9}$ (where X = ° F)

For purposes of mental calculation, remember that between the freezing and boiling points — the range of practical application in hydrotherapy — every 5 ° C is equivalent to 9 ° F and vice versa, and that every 1 ° C is equivalent to 1.8 ° F and vice versa. For purposes of memorization, the most memorable equivalents are:

Centigrade	Fahrenheit
10	50
37	98.6
40	104
60	140
100	212

Knowing these equivalents can quickly orient you from one system of measurement to the other.

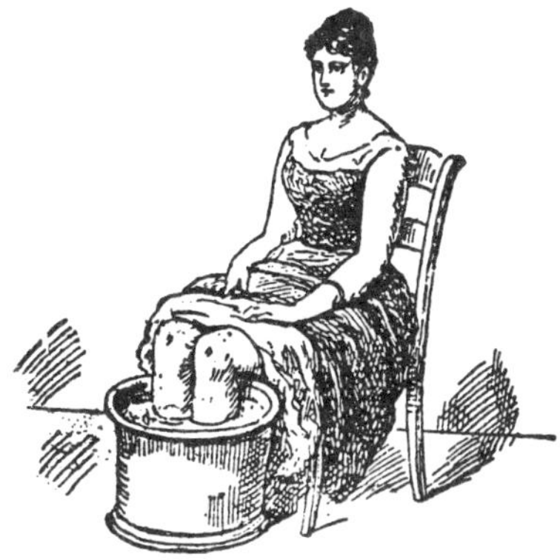

12. DEMONSTRATION: HOT FOOT BATH

INTRODUCTION:

The hot foot bath is one of the simplest and most frequently employed hydrotherapeutic measures. It is often used as part of a more extensive treatment, such as the Russian bath, as we will demonstrate subsequently. It is simple enough that it can easily be prescribed over the phone, when appropriate, as a home treatment.

DEFINITION:

local immersion of feet and ankles in water from 104-110° F (40-43° C) for 10-30 minutes

MATERIALS:

foot tub
bath thermometer
blanket
towels
washcloth
hot water source
chair
pitcher of ice water
mustard powder, if desired

PROCEDURE:

assemble all the above materials
inform patient of the treatment's nature, rationale, duration, cost, etc.
make sure patient is comfortable in regard to position, room temperature, etc.
seat patient on chair
drape patient with blanket (if patient is sensitive to blanket material, drape patient with cotton sheet first)
fill foot tub with water 104° F
add mustard powder, if desired, to intensify treatment
place your hands under the patient's bare feet and guide them into the tub so that your hands enter the water first (this provides a double check on the water temperature)
extend drape so that it covers the tub
over next 5 minutes add hotter water to gradually bring foot bath temperature to 110° F; remove feet before each addition of water to avoid burning
allow bath to continue for a total of 10-30 minutes, as required, monitoring bath temperature and adding hot water, as necessary, to maintain temperature
apply cold compress (a cotton washcloth wrung out in cold water and folded in thirds) to forehead and/or back of neck, as needed, to help prevent/reduce cerebral congestion
at the end of the treatment, remove the feet from the tub and pour cold water briefly over all surfaces of the feet and ankles
dry feet and ankles thoroughly with towel
if patient is perspiring, give a brief witch hazel or alcohol rub
have patient lie down and rest for at least 15 minutes

MECHANISM: (I) 5 min (R)

hot → dilation →↑ flow → stasis →↑ blood to feet → ↓ blood in congested areas = derivation
hot →↑ metabolism →↑ body temperature also comes into play

INDICATIONS:

congestive headache
nosebleed
pulmonary congestion
pelvic congestion
suppressed menstruation
chill
fatigue
preparation for cold treatments
plantar warts

CONTRAINDICATIONS:

peripheral vascular disease
e.g., arteriosclerosis
thromboangiitis obliterans (Buerger's disease)
deep vein thrombosis

why? hot → ↑ metabolism —(↓ vasculature)→ ↓ tissue

this concept is important to understand because it comes into play with every hot treatment to the extremities; permanent tissue damage can result if the impaired vasculature is unable to support the increased metabolism which results from the hot treatment

loss of sensation
why? without sensory feedback the patient may suffer damaging burns unawares

diabetes mellitus
why? ↓ sensation
↓ vasculature
↑ blood glucose

loss of consciousness

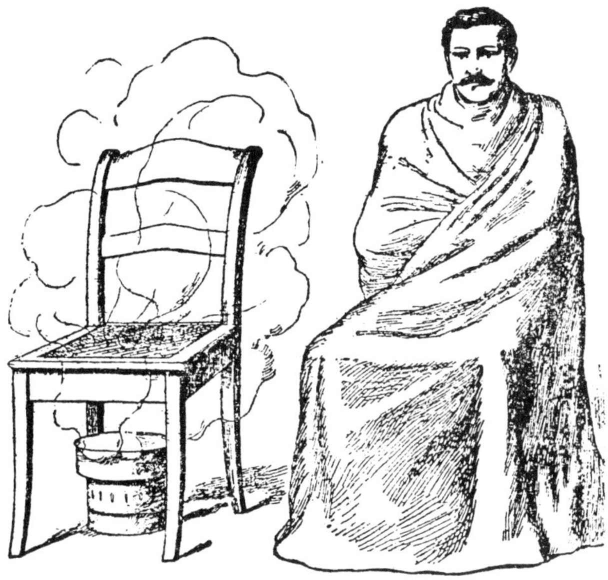

13.DEMONSTRATION: RUSSIAN BATH

INTRODUCTION:

There are a number of portable and permanent Russian bath installations which are much fancier than the home treatment we will now demonstrate, but if you understand the principles and procedures of this makeshift treatment, you will certainly be able to apply this bath successfully with more elaborate equipment.

DEFINITION:

a full-body steam bath excluding the head

MATERIALS:

wooden or plastic chair
tea kettle
hot plate
blankets
towels
hot foot bath (see Chapter 12)
washcloth

oral thermometer
timepiece with second hand
warm drinking water or diaphoretic herb tea (see page 165)
cold shower or equipment for cold mitten friction (see Chapter 26)

PROCEDURE:

assemble above materials
inform patient of treatment's nature, rationale, duration, cost, etc.
make sure patient is comfortable and treatment area is draft-free, etc.
seat disrobed patient on chair
drape patient with two blankets, one from neck to floor in front and one from neck to floor in back

if patient is sensitive to wool, drape patient with cotton sheet first

insert towel around neck inside of blankets to act as seal against steam
take and record pulse and temperature
apply hot foot bath (see Chapter 12)
place hot plate with boiling kettle of water inside blankets and under chair (substitute electric kettle if available)
make sure kettle spout is directed away from patient
make sure hot plate is safely away from blankets or any other flammable material

Take all precautions not to burn the patient or catch anything on fire

allow treatment to go 5-10 minutes for stimulative effects and 15-25 minutes for sedative effects
monitor and record pulse and temperature every 5 minutes
do not allow pulse to exceed 140 or temperature to exceed 104° F
apply and renew cool compresses to forehead as needed

offer appropriate warm drinks such as hot water and herbal teas, e.g., ginger, to patient to maintain hydration and promote diaphoresis

terminate treatment with short cold shower

if a shower is not available, apply cold mitten friction (see Chapter 26) while patient stands in hot foot bath and then terminate foot bath by pouring cold water over feet

have patient lie down and rest well-covered for at least 30 minutes

MECHANISM:

hot —(5-10 min.)→ dilation →↑ flow —(10-15 more min.)→ stasis and tissue relaxation

hot →↑ metabolism →↑ oxidation of toxins
→↑ body temperature →
↑ sweating →
↑ elimination

Note: most of the heat comes from the condensation of the steam rather than from the actual temperature of the steam

INDICATIONS:

colds
flu
chronic intoxication with drugs, alcohol, tobacco or environmental poisons
hypotension
rheumatoid arthritis
insomnia
nervous agitation
congestive headache
sinus congestion
preparation for cold treatments
preparation for massage and/or visceral manipulation
gout
jaundice
prophylaxis in a healthy patient

CONTRAINDICATIONS:

anemia
diabetes
heart disease
hypertension
peripheral vascular disease, e.g., arteriosclerosis
emaciation
weakness or debility

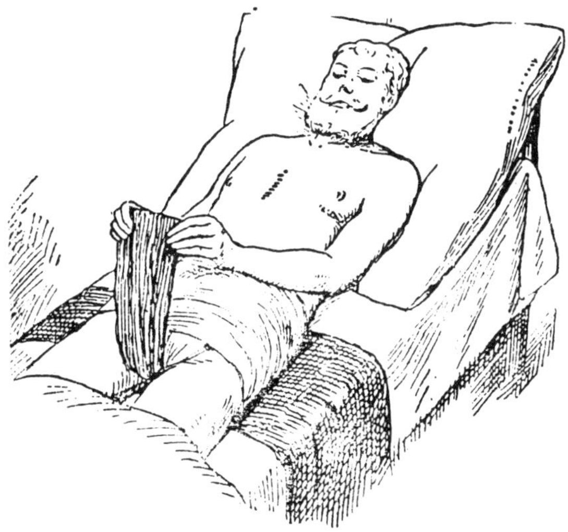

14. DEMONSTRATION: HEATING COMPRESSES

"The history of the use of water as a remedy serves to direct attention to an attitude of the medical profession which still persists, a simple agent such as water, which is cheap and easily available, is often neglected for a complicated system of therapy which is not so effective."

— J. S. Coulter

INTRODUCTION:

Heating compresses are useful, versatile and well-suited to home treatment and prescription over the telephone.

DEFINITION:

moist heat via a cold compress applied to a body part and covered with wool or flannel; (how can a cold application be hot? see page 20 if you don't know the answer)

MATERIALS:

cotton cloth large enough to cover area to be treated
wool or flannel cloth large enough to cover cotton cloth

safety pins or other fastening devices
impervious material if a strong heating effect is desired, e.g., oil cloth or plastic (various sizes of plastic baggies or garbage bags are convenient)
water at desired temperature (usually cold tap water)
towels and blankets, as needed

PROCEDURE:

assemble above materials
inform patient of the nature and rationale of the treatment
make sure patient is comfortable
make sure patient is warm; give hot foot bath, if necessary
wring out cotton compress material in cold water so it does not drip
apply compress to part to be treated (wrist, knee, trunk, etc.)
add impervious covering to increase heating effects, if desired; this is strongly recommended if the patient is weak, chilly, has poor circulation or if it is the first such treatment and you do not know how the patient will respond; if it is a large compress such as a trunk compress, extra blankets can partially substitute for an impervious cover
wrap snuggly in flannel or wool so no air can circulate within the compress; why? air causes excess cooling through evaporation and may increase congestion
but do not wrap so tightly that respiration or blood circulation is hampered
use safety pins, tape, velcro or other fastening device, if necessary to secure wrap
keep compress in place overnight
- or until dry
- or for several hours, then remove and dry the area and renew the compress
- or, if giving a long series of compresses over a considerable length of time, allow one hour of rest in between applications to reduce the risk of dermatitis

end treatment in all cases with a cool friction rub (see Chapter 26)
dry treatment area thoroughly
rest patient
do not allow patient to become chilled
use socks, gloves, hats, shirts, sleeves, sweaters, underwear, etc. as ready-made compresses and coverings, e.g., have the patient suffering the discomfort of a chest cold take a warm shower before retiring, wring out a cotton tee shirt in cold tap water and put it on, then put a wool sweater over that and go to bed for the night with plenty of wool blankets and comforters

MECHANISM:

the cold causes an initial vasoconstriction which is soon followed by vasodilation which leads to a warming of the tissue; as heat builds up within the compress, further dilation results; if an impervious covering has been applied, heat will build up even higher, causing a relaxation of the tissue and a strong derivative effect; if no impervious covering has been applied, cooling gradually takes place due to evaporation which brings with it the results of the initial cool treatment, and the treatment cycles back through the phases already described; a constant, gentle self-modulating treatment has been put in place; we've mentioned vicious cycles which have escaped regulation; this could be described as a beneficial cycle; as heat builds up, evaporation is increased which reduces the heat; as the compress cools, evaporation decreases, allowing the heat to build back up again; this vacillation between the cool and warm temperatures gives a strong tonic effect to the tissues, increasing circulation and decreasing congestion; so think of the impervious covering as resulting in derivative effects and the non-impervious covering as resulting in tonic effects

INDICATIONS:

trunk compress: (may be divided into chest and abdominal compresses)

chest compress:

acute mastitis

chronic bronchitis

pneumonia (if fever is greater than 103 ° F, change compress every half hour)

chest cold

early influenza

cough

asthma; if *acute,* start with *hot first* for 5-10 minutes; if acute and fever is present, grade hot application according to the following:

99-100 ° F : 3 minutes hot

100-101 ° F : 2 minutes hot

101-102 ° F : 1 minute hot

abdominal compress:

constipation

diarrhea

backache (make sure compress goes all the way around to back)

poor digestion

gas

chronic appendicitis

insomnia

Crohn's disease

ulcerative colitis

irritable bowel syndrome

for the above three conditions have patient sleep in pack 5 nights a week for 2 weeks then rest 1 week and repeat

biliary stasis

hepatic torpor

throat compress: (should not be wrapped around neck but rather drawn across the front of the neck from ear-to-ear and fastened on top of the head)

pharyngitis
laryngitis
tonsilitis
lymphadenopathy

other: (as needed over any area)

boils
cellulitis
lymphangitis
pain
arthritis
sprains

CONTRAINDICATIONS:

debilitated patient who cannot react
chilly patient with low body temperature (less than 98 ° F) unless warmed up first by other treatment
over skin conditions irritated by moisture
abdominal compresses with impervious coverings should be used with caution, if at all, in cases of portal congestion

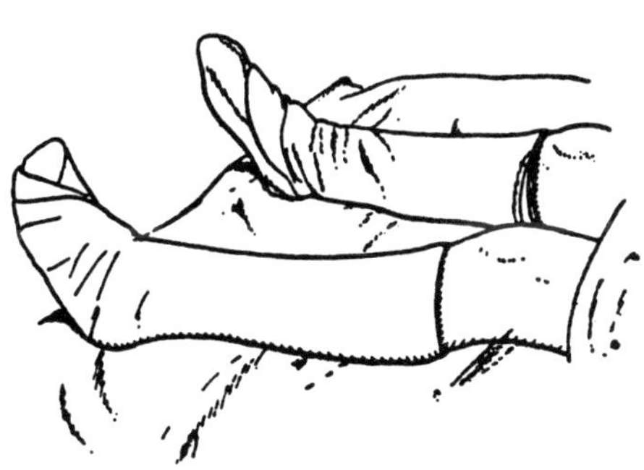

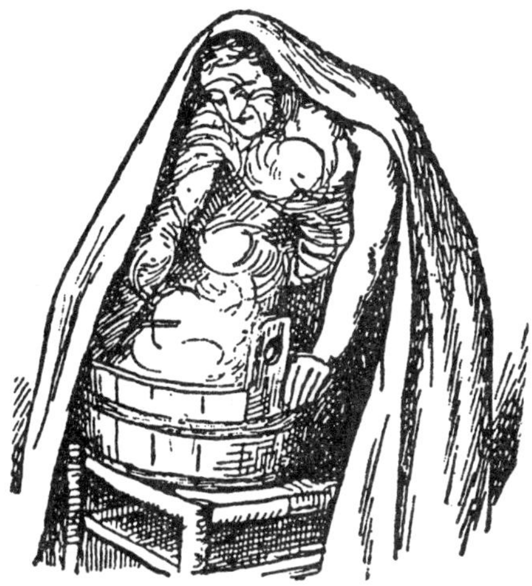

15. DEMONSTRATION: STEAM INHALATION

INTRODUCTION:

What we are about to demonstrate may be obsolete in light of the current availability of inexpensive commercial vaporizers, but if you understand how to apply this makeshift treatment, you will never be at a loss for a steam inhalation treatment whether you have a vaporizer or not.

DEFINITION:

a hot, moist air bath to the respiratory tract

MATERIALS:

tea kettle with boiling water
hot plate
aromatic oils, e.g., eucalyptus (optional)
sheet
umbrella
bedside stand
newspaper funnel

PROCEDURE:

assemble above materials
inform patient as to nature and rationale of treatment
make sure patient is comfortable lying on bed
fill kettle with water and bring to boil
add medicated oils, if desired
place kettle on hot plate and hot plate on bedside stand
with umbrella and sheet rig a "tent" to cover patient's head and kettle
roll a section of newspaper into a large cone
use cone to direct steam toward patient
have patient breath slowly and deeply
Take all precautions not to burn patient and not to set materials on fire
wipe patient's face with cool damp cloth, as necessary
continue treatment for 30-60 minutes, as many as three times per day
at end of treatment dry and rest patient for a half hour

MECHANISM:

expectorations are increased by liquifying the mucus from the respiratory tract with hot, wet air
heating the mucosa via the condensing steam increases circulation to the respiratory tract and decreases congestion
aromatic oils, if used, increase penetration and add their own medicinal effects, such as antisepsis, as well as a pleasant fragrance

INDICATIONS:

cough
laryngitis
respiratory tract congestion
sore throat
spasmodic breathing
dry, thick secretions

CONTRAINDICATIONS:

- extremely young or extremely old patients may not be able to respond properly to the heat
- congestive heart failure (moist air might aggravate already compromised breathing)
- cardiac asthma and other serious heart problems for same reason

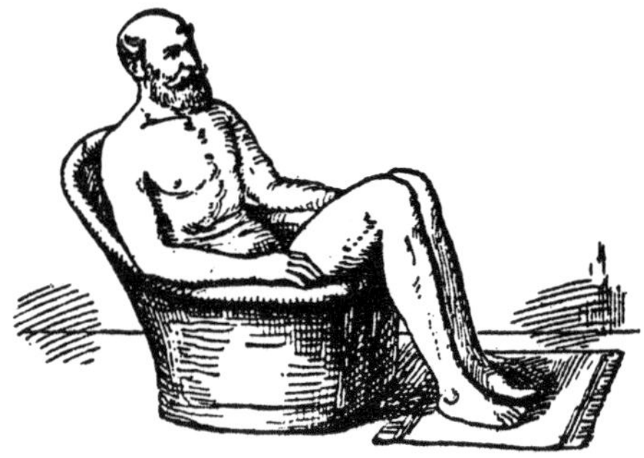

16. DEMONSTRATION: SITZ BATH

INTRODUCTION:

The sitz bath is also called the sitting bath or hip bath. Historically it was one of the mainstays of hydrotherapy, because of its ability to powerfully affect the organs of the lower abdomen and pelvis. Like many hydrotherapies it has fallen into disuse because it is relatively labor-intensive and inconvenient and because its virtues are no longer taught in medical schools. However, with a little ingenuity and effort, this most useful treatment can be made part of any naturopathic practice.

DEFINITION:

an immersion bath with the patient seated in a tub, water covering the hips, buttocks and lower abdomen

MATERIAL:

washtub(s) or sitz tub(s), if available
foot tub
towels
bath thermometer
sheet/blanket to cover patient, if necessary
hot water
cold water
washcloths

PROCEDURE:

assemble above materials
inform patient of nature and rationale of treatment
make sure patient is comfortable
place a towel on bottom of washtub(s) and drape towels over the front and back of the tub(s) to protect patient's buttocks, back and popliteal area
(for patient's convenience in getting up and down, elevate sitz tub on blocks)
fill sitz and foot tubs with water of appropriate temperature and in appropriate amounts as per the following:

	Hot Sitz	Cold Sitz	Neutral Sitz
amount:	½" above navel	½" below navel	to navel
temp:	106-110° F	55-75° F	92-97° F
	(41-43° C)	(12-24° C)	(33-36° C)
foot bath:	110-112° F	105-110° F	—
	(43-45° C)	(40-43° C)	—
duration:	3-8 min.	3-8 min.	¼-2 hours

Alternate hot & cold sitz
2-5 minutes hot
20-60 seconds cold

carefully assist disrobed patient in and out of sitz bath(s)
cover patient with sheet and/or blanket, if necessary
in hot sitz, apply cold compresses to forehead and back of neck
finish hot sitz by pouring cold water over all parts bathed in hot
start alternate sitz with hot and end with cold
finish hot foot bath with cold affusion to feet (see Chapter 12)
dry patient
rest patient lying down for at least a half hour

MECHANISM:

derivation from head and lungs

direct effects according to temperature and time (e.g., hot is relaxing, cold tonifying and neutral calmative)

spinal cord reflexive effects to underlying pelvic and abdominal organs

hot foot bath minimizes possible congestion via derivative effects

INDICATIONS:

Hot	Cold	Alternate	Neutral
painful spasm:	enuresis	vaginal infection	acute cystitis
vaginismus	prolapsus:	*chronic* UTI	excitement:
tenesmus	uterine	pelvic congestion	mental
colic: e.g.,	cystocele	PID	sexual
uterine	rectocele	*improving*	pruritis ani
nephritic	constipation	neuralgias	pruritis vulvae
intestinal	stage fright	improving	
neuralgia:	benign prostatic	insomnia	
ovarian	hypertrophy	hemorrhoids	
testicular	(BPH)	fissures	
intestinal	menorrhagia	prostatitis	
sciatica	incontinence	congestive	
lumbago	due to BPH	headache	
insomnia		constipation	
suppressed menses		postpartum	
congestive			
headache			
painful			
hemorrhoids			

CONTRAINDICATIONS:

Specific:

Hot	Cold	Alternate
hemorrhage	acute inflammation	see listings under hot and cold
menorrhagia	painful conditions	
atonic conditions, e.g., prolapsus	spasms	
pelvic congestion	colics	
	acute lung congestion	
	heart problems	

General:

inability to move with ease and safety (obesity, debility)
hot foot bath is contraindicated in peripheral vascular disease

Please note:

the indications for the cold sitz bath are roughly the same as the contraindications for the hot sitz bath and vice versa: the contraindications for the alternate sitz bath would be a combination of the contraindications for the hot and cold sitz baths; please note that *acute urinary tract infections* (UTI) are treated by *neutral sitz baths only,* while *chronic* urinary tract infections may be given *alternate* sitz baths; strong temperatures, either hot or cold, over a closed, superficial viscus, such as the bladder, which is inflamed, should be avoided, because of the risk of temporarily making an already painful condition even worse.

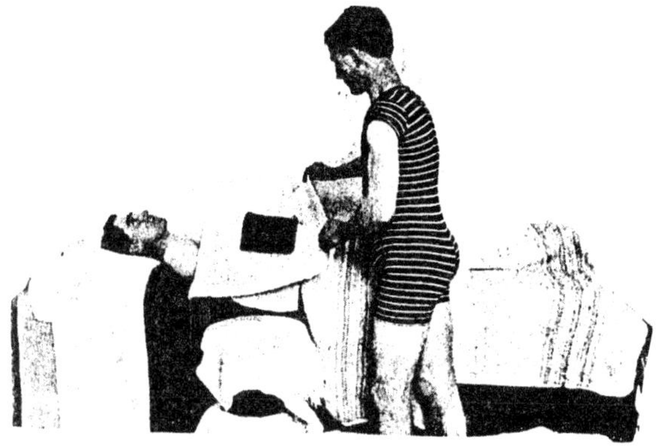

17. DEMONSTRATION: FOMENTATIONS

INTRODUCTION:

Fomentations represent a powerful hydrotherapeutic tool for use in a wide variety of acute conditions.

DEFINITION:

the local application, usually repeated, of moist heat via compresses of wool or other material

MATERIALS:

treatment table
blanket
sheet
pillow
oral thermometer
tub thermometer
materials for hot foot bath (see Chapter 12)
materials for cold mitten friction (see Chapter 26)
tub of very hot water (140-212°) (with mustard powder, 1 T/qt., if desired)
mechanical wringer, if available
washcloths for compresses and friction
towels

wool or flannel fomentation material of appropriate sizes (towels, sponges and hydroculation packs are acceptable)
fomentation packs or other insulating material (towels are acceptable)

PROCEDURE:

assemble above materials
inform patient of nature and rationale of treatment
make sure patient is comfortable
have disrobed patient lay supine on table which has been covered with an open sheet and/or blanket
take and record patient's temperature (pulse too, if it will be an intense treatment over a large body area)
apply hot foot bath (see Chapter 12) (this may be impractical if patient must, for some reason, be in prone position, in which case, use a hot water bottle to the feet)
wring out several thicknesses of fomentation material in very hot water (remember, the more water left in the material, the more heat it possesses)
(if a mechanical wringer, e.g., from an old-fashioned washing machine, is not available, the fomentation should be wet only in the broadest middle area, leaving the ends dry so they may be grasped for wringing out by hand without burning the operator)
insert fomentation in fomentation pack or cover it with several layers of dry toweling (note: it may be applied directed only when much less heat is used)
protect any bony prominences with extra insulation
apply fomentation to indicated area(s)
(note: applications for direct effects would be larger, while reflex applications should be smaller)
close sheet and/or blanket
monitor patient's reactions
if application becomes too hot, remove it briefly and dry the skin and/or add additional insulation material

change the fomentation every 3-10 minutes
between fomentations briefly apply a cold compress or cold friction
apply a cold compress to the forehead or throat by the second fomentation or when perspiration starts
repeat the fomentation 2-3 times
keep hot foot bath at required temperatures
for intense treatments monitor pulse and temperature (don't let pulse go above 140 or temperature go above 104 °F)
after last fomentation finish with whole-body cold mitten friction (Chapter 26)
(note: omit with pleurisy, dysmenorrhea and arthritis or rheumatism aggravated by cold)
wrap patient warmly, rest patient for half an hour
for daily treatments protect patient's skin with vaseline or cocoa butter

MECHANISM:

very hot → constriction → dilation → derivation →↓ congestion
→↑ metabolism
→↑ sweat →↑ elimination
→ tissue relaxation →↓ spasm →↓ pain

INDICATIONS:

in general: PAIN, CONGESTION, INFLAMMATION
muscle tension, spasm, soreness
insomnia
preparation for cold treatment, massage or manipulation
bronchitis, pleurisy, chest colds
sciatica, lumbago, intercostal neuralgia
boils (to bring to a head)
dysmenorrhea
gallstones
renal colic
cardiac collapse from drugs

ovaritis
prostatitis
nephritis
gastroenteritis

CONTRAINDICATIONS:

see hot foot bath (Chapter 12)
see cold mitten friction (Chapter 26)
myocardial infarction
vascular disease of extremities including diabetes mellitus
malignancy
hemorrhage
gastric ulcers
loss of sensation

Note: Take precautions not to burn or blister patient

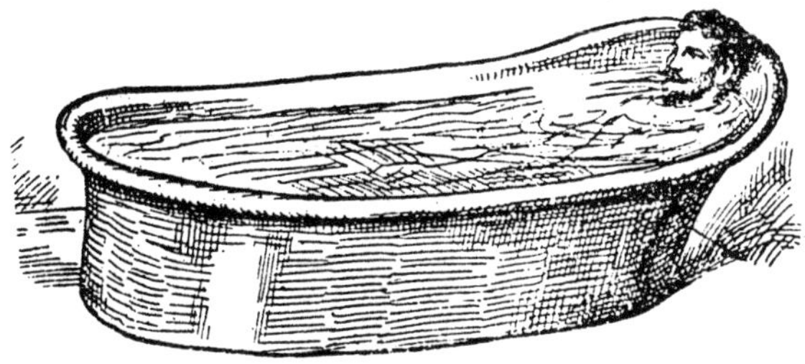

18. DEMONSTRATION: NEUTRAL BATH

INTRODUCTION:

The neutral bath, sometimes called the continuous bath, is a non-thermic hydrotherapy of great value. It was used for years in mental hospitals as a sedative to disturbed patients. Recent studies show it is effective in toxemia of pregnancy because of its reflex action on the kidneys.

DEFINITION:

whole-body immersion in water approximately 92-97° F

MATERIALS:

full-size bathtub
bath thermometer
towels
air pillow
sheet

PROCEDURE:

assemble above materials
inform patient as to nature and rationale of treatment
make sure room is comfortable
fill full-size bathtub with water of neutral temperature (see page 29)
assist disrobed patient into tub
make patient comfortable with pillow or rolled towel for head

adjust water to a temperature neutral to patient
- patient should feel somewhere between "comfortably warm" and neither warm nor cold; this is a better guide than the thermometer in most patients, although the actual water temperature should be monitored, in any case

cover any exposed parts, e.g., knees, with towels, or cover whole tub with sheet

patient should be relaxed and quiet

lighting should be dim

add water, as necessary, to maintain neutral temperature

duration: ¼-1 hour for insomnia
- up to 3-4 hours in fever and mania
- Note: if a treatment of greater than 4 hours is planned, the patient's skin should be rubbed ahead of time with lanolin
- (in the past, baths lasting days and even weeks were employed with benefit; in such cases the patient was removed from the bath every 3 hours to use the toilet and to have oil applied to the skin)

cool water a few degrees at the end of the treatment

assist patient out of tub

dry quickly but gently without friction which would be too stimulating for a calmative treatment

rest patient for half an hour

MECHANISM:

neutral temperature → equalization of circulation → ↓ congestion → sedation (if cerebral congestion exists)

neutral temperature = "physiological zero" = it shuts off nervous input and output and therefore → tranquilization and nerve restoration

kidney function is increased probably through a reflex stimulation from the skin as well as hydrostatic pressure on vascular system from the bath

INDICATIONS:

insomnia
nervous exhaustion
anxiety
depression
mental illness
when hot or cold is contraindicated
e.g., diabetes, arteriosclerosis
fever
acute hypertension
intractable itching
chronic, intractable pain
toxemia of pregnancy
peripheral edema
drug withdrawal
cleansing or healing crisis

CONTRAINDICATIONS:

eczema or other skin condition aggravated by water
great cardiac weakness

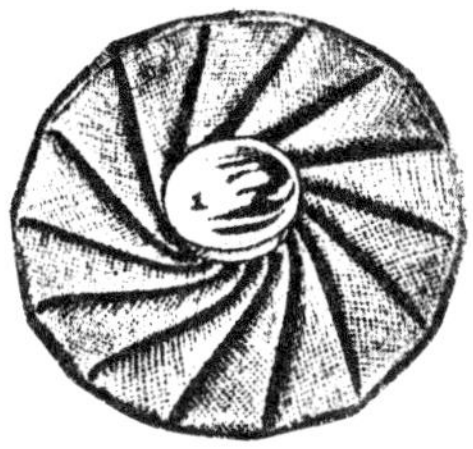 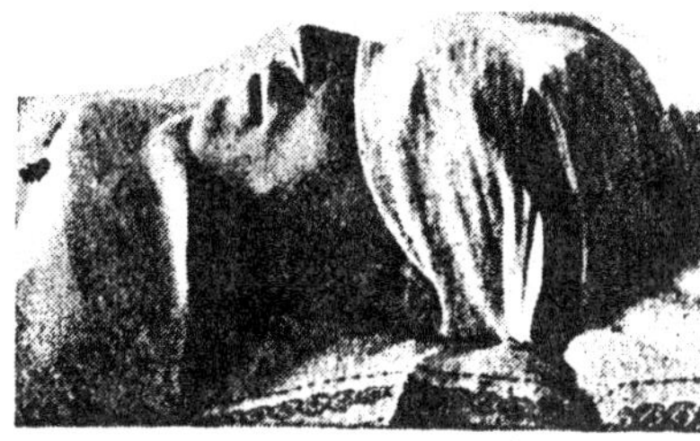

19. DEMONSTRATION: ICE PACK

INTRODUCTION:

Everyone is familiar with the ice pack, if only from cartoons and movies which depict hungover revelers with icebags on their heads or assault victims using cold steaks to soothe their black eyes. There are many other uses for ice packs, but they are based on the same principles which make the above examples effective. There are a number of ready-made cold packs available in various sizes and shapes for convenient application, but we will demonstrate a "homemade" pack from everyday household materials.

DEFINITION:

local application of ice over a protected body part

MATERIALS:

flannel big enough to cover treatment area
towels
safety pins
plastic
crushed ice

PROCEDURE:

assemble above materials
inform patient of nature and rationale of treatment

make sure patient is comfortably situated
spread towel flat and spread crushed ice one inch thick over an area large enough to cover lesion
fold and pin towel so ice stays securely in place
cover treatment area with flannel
place ice pack over flannel
place sheet of plastic over ice pack
place towel or bandage over plastic to hold it and ice pack securely in place (an elastic bandage is very good for this)
place another sheet of plastic over this to protect bedding and clothing
leave pack in place for at least 15, but not more than 30, minutes
remove pack
observe and note reaction
cover treatment area
repeat ice pack every 1 to 3 hours, as needed

MECHANISM:

long cold → constriction → dilation → constriction → ↓ circulation (retrostasis) →↓ swelling →↓ congestion (depletion)
long cold →↓ metabolism
→↓ pain
Note: cold is generated from the melting ice which absorbs 80 times more heat than water does

INDICATIONS:

sprains
contusions
acute bursitis
acute joint inflammation (except when aggravated by cold)
tennis elbow
toothache
headache (also as ice collar to abort migraines)
goiter
hemorrhage (remember reflex areas)

acute appendicitis
inflamed hemorrhoids
impending hemorrhagic stroke (as ice collar)
tachycardia in prolonged hot treatment
fever
anorexia (over stomach before meals)
cerebral congestion
insect bites including brown recluse spider bites and centipede bites
after dental surgery

CONTRAINDICATIONS:

acute asthma (over lungs)
acute cystitis (over bladder)
in patients aggravated by cold
in patients averse to, or afraid of, cold

Note: Dr. Carroll considered ice therapy "unphysiological" and never used it. Drs. Dick and Scott, likewise, do not favor ice packs, finding them unnecessary and suppressive.

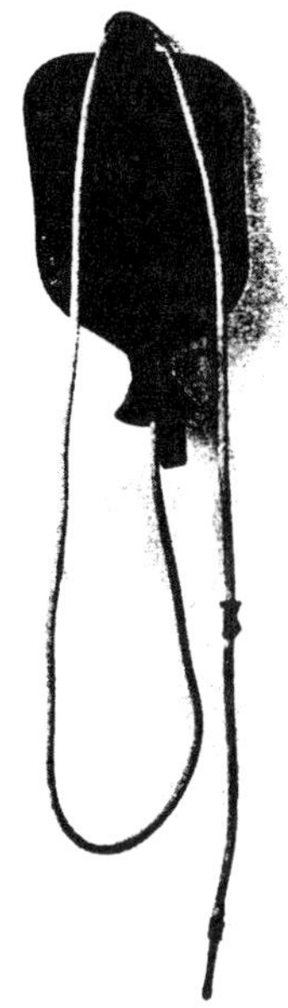

20. ENEMAS

We will make numerous references to enemas for the management of various conditions. There are many schools of thought concerning the proper techniques for administering enemas. We will give a brief summary of a method for applying enemas we have found useful.

The enema can be used for cases of inflammation, congestion and/or pain anywhere in the body, especially when the bowels are not moving. The rectum has reflex relationships throughout the body. When it is distended naturally with feces and flatus or experimentally with gauze, a multitude of diffuse symptoms may be elicited or aggravated. Enemas are effective against pain and inflammation because they eliminate irritating toxins from the body and because they relieve rectal distention and its painful reflex effects.

Procedure for administering an enema

make sure patient is well hydrated so enema solution will not be absorbed out of the bowel

have patient lay supine with knees flexed
elevate buttocks with a pillow protected by plastic
to prevent cramping and retention select water temperature according to oral temperature of patient as per the following:

Oral Temperature	Enema Temperature
95° F	110° F
96	108
97	106
98.6	105
99	104
100	103
101	101
102	102
103	103
104	104

use water only, except in the following cases:
colic in an infant — mild infusion of catnip or chamomile may be used
acute intoxication such as snake bite, drug overdose, poisoning, or renal failure — add activated charcoal
infestation (pinworms) — quassia bark infusion may be added
impaction — Castile soap or olive oil may be added
ulcerative colitis — golden seal may be added
bowel irritation with chronic diarrhea — corn starch may be added
pain of malignancy — coffee may be added
fill enema bag with appropriate amount of enema solution
- adults: 1-2 quarts depending on size
- infants (less than 1 year): 2-6 oz. (use 1-3 bulbfuls of a 2-oz. bulb syringe)
- 1-2 year-olds: 6-12 oz.
- 3-4 year-olds: 12-16 oz.
- 5-10 year-olds: 16-32 oz.

bleed air from enema tube

lubricate nozzle with oil or vaseline
insert nozzle gently into rectum toward navel
fix enema bag 10-30 inches above patient according to how quickly you wish the fluid to enter (the lower the bag, the lower the hydrostatic pressure and, therefore, the slower the entry of the solution)
release solution through tube, adjusting water pressure, as necessary, by changing the height of the bag or by manually compressing the tube
if patient feels bulging or pressure in the abdomen, stop and wait patiently; do not push the bulge; it may take 5 minutes, but it should naturally subside; if pressure remains, have patient gently massage area where pressure is felt; deep breathing may also be helpful
once patient has accepted as much enema solution as practical, have patient retain it for as long as possible — up to 15-20 minutes — then evacuate and rest

Note: Enemas should not be abused. Enemas are remedial, not preventative or strengthening. Reserve their use for well-indicated clinical situations.

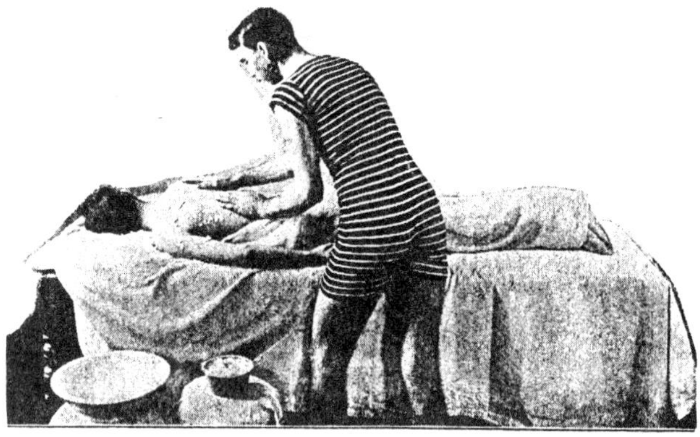

21. DEMONSTRATION: SALT GLOW

INTRODUCTION:

Like most hydrotherapies the salt glow is a labor-intensive treatment which well rewards its users. It holds a special place in the hydrotherapeutic armamentarium, along with the neutral bath, because it does not necessarily rely on thermic impressions.

DEFINITION:

a friction application of wet salt rubbed on the skin

MATERIALS:

2-4 pounds of coarse salt (Epsom salts are excellent, although table salt will do)
basin
stool or chair
hot foot bath (see Chapter 12)
towels
sheet
blanket
water source to remove salt from body (tub, spray, shower, affusion, etc.)

PROCEDURE:

assemble above materials
inform patient as to the nature and rationale of treatment
make sure patient is comfortable
seat disrobed patient on a stool (ideally in a large bathtub)
drape patient with sheet and then blanket
apply hot foot bath (see Chapter 12)
wet salt to a sticky consistency (do not dissolve)
expose part to be treated
wet skin
rub a handful of moistened salt on skin with back-and-forth friction until skin turns pink or to tolerance
Note: dark-complexioned people generally tolerate vigorous applications better than the fair-complexioned
do arms first, starting with fingers
do legs next, starting with toes
then do in order: chest, abdomen, back, hips and buttocks
remove salt by spray, shower, bath or affusion using water of a cool but pleasant temperature
rub skin during the rinse
dry with vigorous friction
rest patient for 30 minutes

MECHANISM:

friction → vasodilation →↑ circulation (w/ no temp △)
chem irritation → dilation →↑ circulation (w/ no temp△)
mechanical/chemical irritation →↑ nerve activity
→↑ sebaceous activity
→↑ skin elimination
this is a tonic hydrotherapy which does not necessarily rely on hot or cold
Note: for an intensified reaction in a strong patient salt may be softened in ice water
Note: Dr. Eli G. Jones claimed that much of the beneficial effect of an Epsom salt glow resulted from the patient's absorption of magnesium through the skin

INDICATIONS:

- chronic conditions, especially those with inactive skin, such as
  - chronic indigestion
  - kidney disease
  - diabetes (only if there are no skin lesions)
- sluggish circulation, especially in those who do not react well to hot or cold
- low vital force
- poor resistance
- frequent colds
- general weakness
- neurasthenia
- epilepsy
- cancer (but not over a palpable tumor)
- locally followed by peanut or other oil for joint problems (see page 199)

CONTRAINDICATIONS:

- skin lesions such as eczema
- friable skin, as, e.g., in Cushing's disease
- same as for hot foot bath (see Chapter 12)
- too frequent treatment may cause skin irritation
- while salt glow may be administered to someone laying on a table, the difficulties of rinsing such a patient make this treatment generally impractical for those who cannot stand or sit
- while not contraindicated, per se, in acute disease, it is, in Kellogg's words, "rarely used"

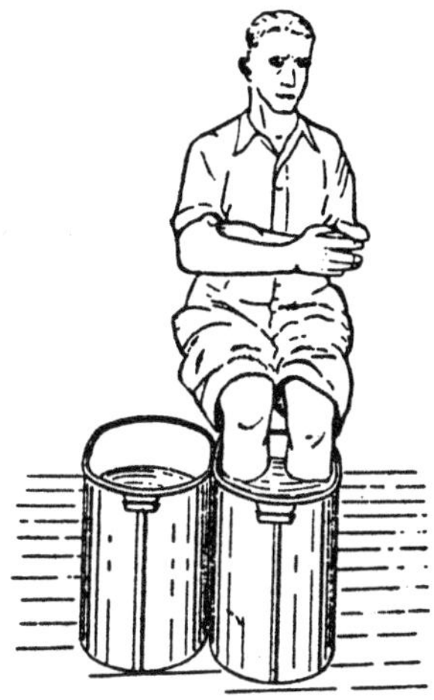

22. DEMONSTRATION: ALTERNATE BATHS

INTRODUCTION:

This is one of the simplest yet most powerful hydrotherapies. It is especially suited as a home treatment for injuries and infections of the extremities.

DEFINITION:

series of immersions of a body part alternately in hot and cold water

MATERIALS:

2 basins or tubs of a size appropriate to the part to be treated
bath thermometer
towels
hot water
cold water (with ice if desired)
disinfectant such as betadyne, vinegar, *Hypericum* tincture, *Calendula* tincture or hydrogen peroxide for an open wound
timepiece with a second hand

PROCEDURE:

assemble above materials

inform patient as to nature and rationale of treatment

make sure patient is comfortable

fill first basin with hot water of approximately 103° F

add vinegar, betadyne, *Hypericum* tincture, hydrogen peroxide or other disinfectant for a septic wound, *Calendula* tincture for an uninfected wound

place part to be treated in this hot water for 3 minutes

fill second basin with cold water between 40 and 70° F; ice may be used for an intensified effect in a vital patient

take treated part out of hot and place directly in cold water for 30 seconds

add hot water to first basin to raise its temperature to 105° F

place treated part directly back into hot water for another 3 minutes

follow this again with 30 seconds cold

repeat this series of alternate hot and cold baths up to a total of from 4-8 sequences, increasing the temperature of the hot bath a couple of degrees each time up to 110° F; do not exceed this temperature, but once it has been achieved, do not let the hot bath fall below it

the duration, number and temperature of the treatments are all variable and should be adjusted appropriately to the individual case

remember, the greater the contrast between the hot and cold baths, the stronger the treatments

also remember that with each alternation the intensity of the reaction is decreased so that after 6-8 sequences a point of diminishing returns is approached

always finish with the short cold bath except in a rheumatoid arthritis patient whose condition is greatly aggravated by cold

dry the treated part thoroughly and do not allow it to be chilled

rest patient for ½ hour

Note: for anatomical parts not easily accommodated by a local bath, e.g., shoulder, neck or side, this technique may be applied by soaking towels or flannel in the water or solution used and applying locally, covering with wool

MECHANISM:

short hot → dilation —short cold→ constriction → dilation → pumping action → ↑ circulation → ↑ removal of toxic products of infection → ↑ healing

short hot → ↑ metabolism

short cold → ↑ metabolism
→ ↑ nutrition
→ ↑ immunity

INDICATIONS:

- infections:
  - lymphangitis
  - cellulitis
  - ingrown toenails
- injuries:
  - sprains (after 24 hours)
  - strains (after 24 hours)
  - bruises (after 24 hours)
  - fractures
- arthritis
- venous stasis ulcers
- edema
- chilblains

CONTRAINDICATIONS:

- cancer
- vascular disease, including diabetes
- diminished sensation
- hemorrhage

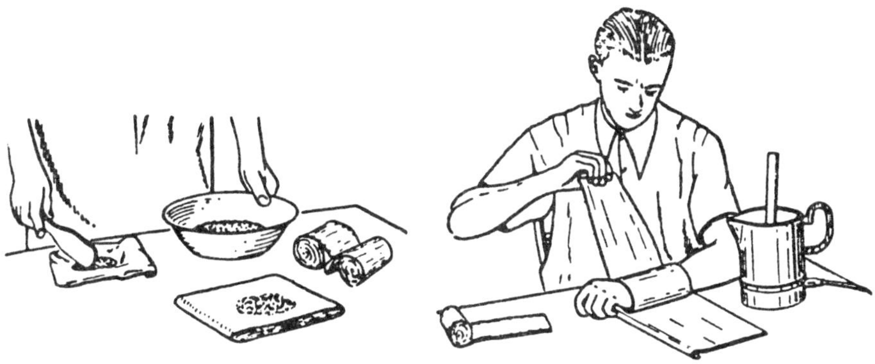

23. DEMONSTRATION: POULTICES

INTRODUCTION:

Poultices combine the local effects of compresses with those of herbal or other beneficial substances.

DEFINITION:

a hot, soft, moist mass of material applied directly to the skin and covered with cotton, then plastic, then wool. It may also be applied between layers of cotton cloth

MATERIALS:

poultice substance, e.g., powdered charcoal, herbs, mustard, clay, coffee or shredded carrots, potatoes, etc.
hot water sufficient to make a paste out of the poultice material (not necessary with freshly shredded vegetables which provide their own moisture)
cotton cloth large enough to cover treatment area
plastic large enough to cover cotton
wool large enough to cover plastic
pin, tape or bandage material for fastening
washcloth
towel

PROCEDURE:

assemble above materials
inform patient as to nature and rationale of treatment
make sure patient is comfortable
moisten poultice material with hot water to make a paste
apply paste to cotton cloth or directly to skin, as convenient, or between layers of cotton, as indicated
Note: for shredded vegetables, no water is added; shredded vegetables are most effectively applied within layers of cheese cloth
place cotton cloth over treatment area
cover with plastic
cover with wool
fasten securely
leave on ½ - 8 hours
remove
clean off all poultice material
apply cold mitten friction(see Chapter 26), if appropriate
dry
cover with clothing or dry bandage

MECHANISM:

short hot → dilation →↑ circulation
after this the application becomes, for all practical purposes, a heating compress with the same mechanism of action. Please see the explanation for this in Chapter 14. Beyond this is the local reaction to the poultice material which, depending on the material(s) used, may include any of the following:
counterirritation
osmotic pull
toxin absorption
astringence
emollience

INDICATIONS:

pain
congestion
inflammation
bee stings
insect bites
abscesses (to bring to a head)
swelling
wound healing
antisepsis

CONTRAINDICATIONS:

allergy to poultice material
condition made worse by poultice, e.g., increasing pus from a wound treated with a poultice

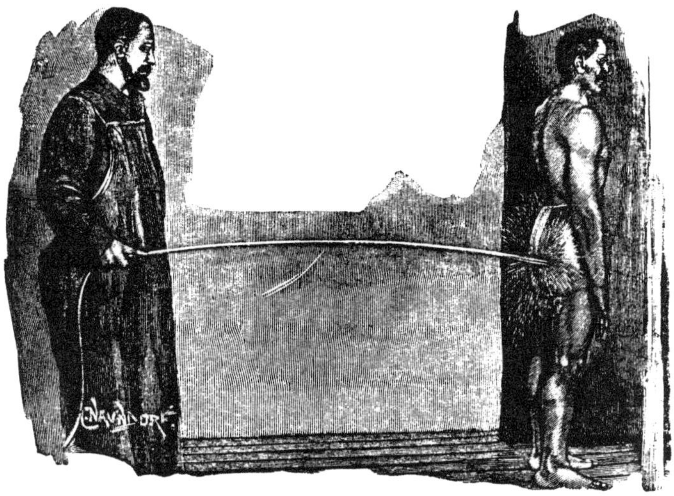

24. DEMONSTRATION: *BLITZ GUSS*

INTRODUCTION:

Historically douches have played a major role in clinical hydrotherapy. Because they require a specially tiled and drained treatment area, they are not always practical today. We will demonstrate only one douche called the "Blitz guss" or "Lightning bath." This was a favorite of Father Kneipp, and was a frequently used treatment first thing in the morning at Lindlahr's sanitarium. It can be done outside in warm weather with a nozzled garden hose. For more information on other douches such as the percussion douche, Scotch douche, rain douche, fan douche, fog douche, etc., please see Kellogg's *Rational Hydrotherapy.*

DEFINITION:

a cold douche to the back of the body starting from the feet up (a reminder: a douche is a stream of water directed against a part of the body or into a body cavity)

MATERIALS:

douche apparatus *or* garden hose with nozzle
cold water source (plus warm water source which can be blended with cold, if available)
towels
warm environment

PROCEDURE:

assemble above materials

inform patient as to nature and rationale of treatment

make sure patient is comfortable, warm and not exposed to chilling drafts or breezes

stand disrobed patient 10-20 feet from water source with back to operator

apply strong water stream (10-60 pounds per square inch) to patient's right foot

move stream promptly up right leg to right buttock

bring stream back down right leg to right foot

apply stream to left foot

move stream promptly up left leg to left buttock

move stream over to right buttock

move stream up right side of back to right shoulder

bring stream back down right side of back to right buttock

move stream over to left buttock

move stream up left side of back to left shoulder

stop stream

the above sequence is illustrated in the following diagram (Figure 6) with numbered arrows on a stick figure:

FIGURE 6

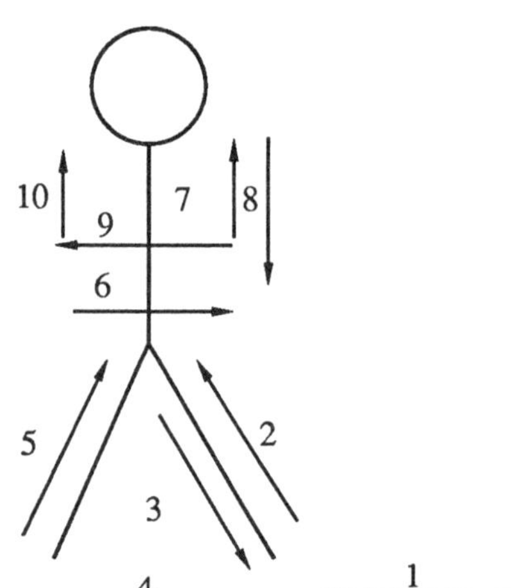

repeat spray sequence up to 5-10 times, as indicated

if hot water is available to blend with the cold, start the first application at a warm temperature and gradually make each repetition colder

if only cold water is available, make sure patient is warm before starting the treatment

how cold to make the douche is graded to the vitality and tolerance of the patient

how quickly to move the douche is graded to the temperatures — the warmer the water, the slower the water stream is moved; the colder the water, the faster the water stream is moved (if a 45 ° F douche were being applied to a vital patient, each spray might last as little as 10-15 seconds

dry patient

rest patient

MECHANISM:

short cold → constriction → dilation $\xrightarrow{\text{repeated}}$ ↑ circulation
↑ metabolism
↑ nutrition
↑ immunity
↑ waste removal

repeated pressure →↑ circulation
→↓ sense of cold →↑ treatment tolerance

INDICATIONS:

neurasthenia

congestion, e.g.,

- liver
- spleen
- bowels

atonic conditions, e.g.,

- dyspepsia
- hypopepsia

constipation
hypothyroidism (with gradual training to colder temperatures)
anemia
alcoholism
drug addiction
to conclude a hot treatment, such as a Russian bath
chronic rheumatism (with gradual training to colder temperatures)

CONTRAINDICATIONS:

acute inflammations, e.g.,
- nephritis
- gastritis
- hepatitis
- sciatica

acute nervous irritability
acute rheumatism
heart disease
hypertension
hyperthyroidism
arteriosclerosis
skin eruptions
severe disease or debility
over bony prominences in thin subjects

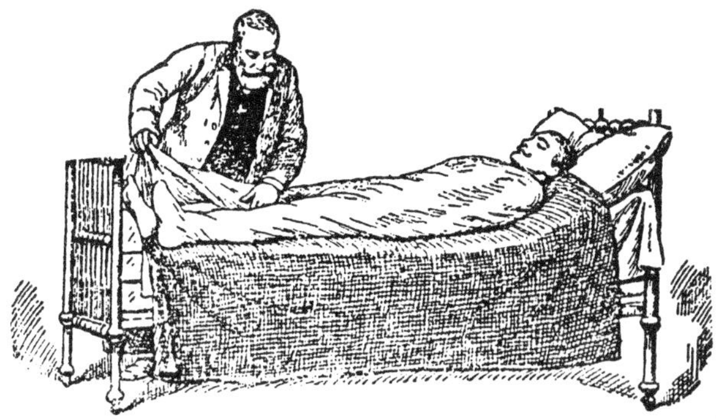

25. DEMONSTRATION: WET SHEET PACK

"If Vincent Priessnitz had never done anything else for mankind but to have discovered and brought into use this form of bath [wet sheet pack], he would have done enough to make him immortal."

— James C. Jackson

INTRODUCTION:

Next to Dr. Carroll's constitutional treatment the wet sheet pack is the most important hydrotherapeutic measure we will discuss. It is an old and reliable treatment. It is powerful, convenient and flexible with a wide, if not universal, application. It is often called the Universal Wet Sheet Pack.

DEFINITION:

a full-body wrap with a cold, wet sheet on the inside and a series of dry blankets on the outside to regulate temperature and evaporation; it amounts to a heating compress to the whole body

MATERIALS:

treatment table
hot foot bath or other warming measure
washcloth for cold compress
2 or more wool blankets
2 large cotton sheets

cold water
towels
pillow
hot packs or infrared lamp, as necessary
friction mitt or terry washcloth

PROCEDURE:

assemble above materials
inform patient of the nature and rationale of the treatment
have patient empty bladder
make sure patient is comfortable
apply hot foot bath or other warming measure, e.g., hot shower, heat lamp, exercise, etc. (Priessnitz used to do these treatments in the morning before his patients rose from the warmth of their beds)
lay pillow at head of table
fold first sheet in quarters lengthwise and lay it lengthwise across the upper part of the table at the bottom of the pillow lopsided fashion so that the long end is on the side of the table away from you and the short end is on your side (leave about 2 feet on your side)
spread first blanket out in a proper lengthwise fashion a few inches below the first sheet and lopsided opposite the first sheet, i.e., toward you
spread second blanket in a similar fashion but lopsided in the other direction, i.e., away from you (in the same direction as the first sheet)
dip second sheet (must be at least as long as patient) in cool water and wring out as dry as possible; two people are needed to do this properly, one on each end
spread wet sheet slightly off center toward you
have nude patient lay down with shoulders a few inches below the top of the wet sheet (in supine position)
note: from this point, work fast to avoid chilling patient
have patient raise both arms above head

pull the far side of the wet sheet over the patient's body but only over the leg on that side

have patient put arms back down at side

pull near (long) side of wet sheet over body and the leg on that side

tuck sheet in and smooth out so that there is maximum contact between the skin and the sheet with no air pockets

close the second blanket, short side first, and wrap patient up mummy style, paying special attention to the neck, making it fit tightly enough so that no air is admitted but loosely enough so that there is no pressure on the blood vessels of the neck

close the first blanket in a similar fashion, tucking long end of the blanket under the patient, if possible

fold both blankets under at the feet but not too tightly, or cramps might result

finish wrap with the long end of the first sheet wrapped around shoulders and tucked around the neck so as to protect the face from the wool blankets

apply hot water bottles, small hydroculator packs or infrared lamp to the feet, as necessary, to insure that they stay warm

apply cold compresses to head, as necessary

offer drinks, as appropriate

Note: the pack can now be taken to four different stages depending on the clinical situation; these stages are explained in the following chart:

STAGES OF THE WET SHEET PACK

Stage:

First (Cooling)	Second (Neutral)	Third (Heating)	Fourth (Sweating)

Duration:

from chilly to not chilly 5-20 min.	not chilly to hot ¼-1 hour	hot to sweating ½-1 hour	sweating to termination 1-2 hours or more

Note: stages can be prolonged by opening blankets or shortened by adding blankets

MECHANISM:

Cold → constriction → dilation →	↑ heat →	↑ dilation →↑ heat →	sweat → elimination
Conduction →↓ heat	97° F = Neutral → sedation	→↑ circulation →↑ derivation →↓ congestion →↑ metabolism →↑ elimination	continue and intensify

General Effects:

tonic, alterative	sedative	stimulative	detoxifying

STAGES OF THE WET SHEET PACK

Stage:

First (Cooling)	Second (Neutral)	Third (Heating)	Fourth (Sweating)

INDICATIONS:

First (Cooling)	Second (Neutral)	Third (Heating)	Fourth (Sweating)
anemia	depression	Crohn's disease	alcohol addiction
weakness	mania	malabsorption	drug addiction
fever	insomnia	nephritis (acute)	nicotine addiction (will stain sheet brown)
convalescense	restlessness	liver congestion	obesity
inability to take bath	melancholy	sinus congestion	measles (to bring out rash)
	neurasthenia	constipation	scarlet fever (to bring out rash)
	anxiety	pneumonia	flu
	delerium	prep for cold treatment	cold
	nervousness	irritable bowel syndrome	bronchitis
	hysteria	ulcerative colitis	jaundice in a strong person
	fever		environmental intoxication
	epilepsy		preventive cleansing
	nervous indigestion		

Special Considerations:

First (Cooling)	Second (Neutral)	Third (Heating)	Fourth (Sweating)
for fever use 2 wet sheets and renew as needed	patient may fall asleep, especially if febrile	string out with cold compress or open blankets	give sip of fluid every 10 min. or 4 oz. every 30 min.
may open pack for cold mitten friction and close back up	don't let patient sleep beyond intended phase		may use diaphoretic teas
anxious patients may get worse in first few minutes but should calm down	if chill occurs, stop treatment and give hot shower		may use extra blankets

Discontinue treatment in any stage if vertigo, headache, restlessness or intolerance, etc., occur

CONTRAINDICATIONS:

Specific:

the heating and sweating stages are contraindicated in anemia

General:

chilled patient (warm up first)
extreme debility (may leave legs and/or arms out of pack in weaker patients)
acute asthma (cover chest with dry cloth)
claustrophobia or fear of treatment (leaving arms out of sheet may help)
skin conditions made worse by moisture
weak heart
severe colds and flu
diabetes or other circulatory problems

Finish:

give cold mitten friction (see Chapter 26) when treatment is terminated regardless of phase completed, but grade the cold mitten friction according to the last phase completed, e.g., that following the heating stage would be stronger than that following the neutral stage

rest patient for ½ hour in dry bedding

Note: this treatment is not so powerful as the constitutional treatment, because it is done without electrical stimulation; however, it is still a potent treatment and capable, in a series, of bringing on a healing crisis

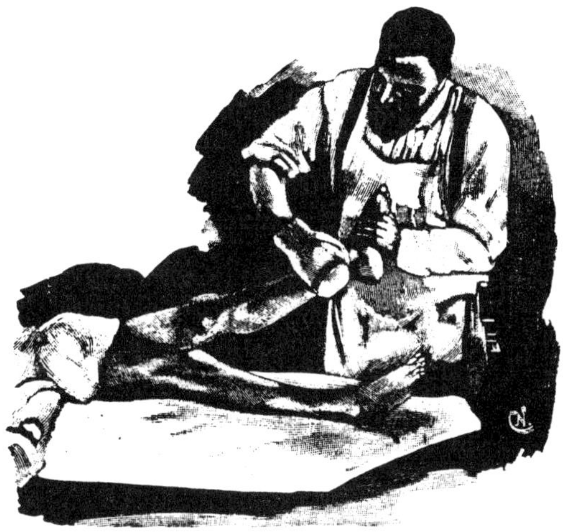

26. DEMONSTRATION: COLD MITTEN FRICTION

INTRODUCTION:

Cold mitten friction is a simple treatment with strong tonic effects which has many uses.

DEFINITION:

cold water ablution with friction from towels, mitts, terry washcloths or loofah

PROCEDURE:

assemble above materials
inform patient of nature and rationale of treatment
make sure patient is comfortable
have nude patient lie supine on blanket, then cover
note: the patient must be warm first
expose and friction only one part at a time, starting with the arm
place dry towel under arm to protect blanket
dip mitt or washcloth in cold water and wring out graded to patient, i.e., drier for a weaker patient
if using washcloth, fold it in half and wrap it around fingers and hold in place with thumb to simulate mitt

using to-and-fro motion, start at the fingers and work up to the shoulders and back to the fingers until the skin becomes pink

redip mitt as necessary

dry arm with friction and cover arm

treat the other arm in the same manner

expose chest and abdomen, keeping arms covered (this is more important in a weak patient)

give to-and-fro friction with a freshly dipped and wrung mitt up the middle of the chest, across to the shoulders, down the sides and back over the midline

may have patient breathe deeply if desired to distract from possible discomfort

repeat and dry and cover

care should be taken to avoid injury to breasts in women and nipples in both sexes

do legs in the same manner as the arms (one at a time, towel under the limb, dry and cover)

have patient turn to the prone position

place pillow under chest, if necessary, and have arms raised to head level

expose back and hips (not legs and arms) and apply friction as done in other areas

dry and cover

rest patient for ½ hour

Note: this was whole-body cold mitten friction, but this treatment can be used locally too

Note: the following variables may be adjusted to fit the clinical situation

- the more forceful the friction (the harder the pressure, the rougher the material), the stronger the reaction
- the lower the temperature, the stronger the reaction
- the more frequent the dipping, the wetter the mitt, the lower the temperature, and therefore the stronger the reaction

in a series of treatments the strength of the treatment may be gradually increased as the patient becomes accustomed to them

MECHANISM:

short cold causes initial vasoconstriction followed quickly by vasodilation which increases the superficial circulation and the elimination of heat and results in a decrease in visceral congestion; at the same time the number and activity of the red and white blood cells is increased, tissue tone is enhanced and metabolism is stimulated resulting in increased heat production and toxin breakdown; the friction, of course, adds greatly to the vasodilatory effects

INDICATIONS:

to finish hot treatments, e.g., wet sheet pack taken to the heating or sweating stage, sauna, jacuzzi, Russian bath, fomentation
cold and flu prevention
poor circulation
anemia
alcohol, drug or tobacco withdrawal
poor resistance to infection
low energy
nervous exhaustion
fever (especially high fever in those unable to tolerate the Brand bath)
anorexia
coma
depression
weak person with infection

CONTRAINDICATIONS:

chilled patient
skin lesions
intolerance to treatment

III.
CONSTITUTIONAL APPROACH

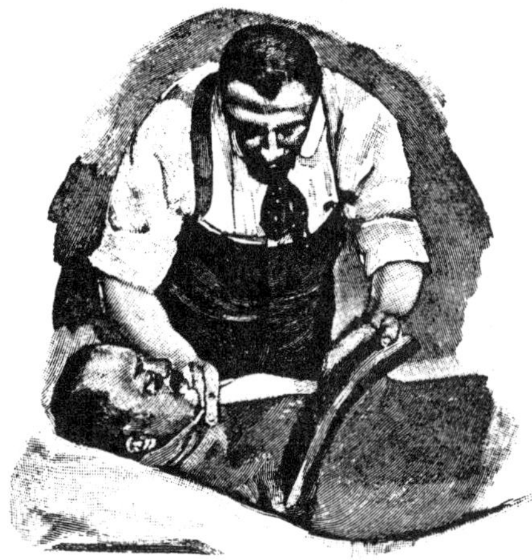

27. DEMONSTRATION: CONSTITUTIONAL TREATMENT

"Discover what will destroy life, and you are a great man, — what will prolong it, and you are an imposter."

— Bulwer

INTRODUCTION:

Constitutional hydrotherapy, as developed and perfected by Dr. O. G. Carroll and his followers, is the most important treatment we will cover in this course.It has been used with wonderful success in a wide variety of conditions for over 60 years. It enhances the immune response, improves overall nutrition, promotes detoxification and helps restore nervous equilibrium. Because it is such a versatile treatment, it is understandable that elder statesmen of its use, such as Dr. Dick, feel that it makes many of the other treatments we have demonstrated unnecessary or obsolete. Compared to the previously discussed treatments, constitutional hydrotherapy is fairly complex. The mechanics of the treatment can only be mastered through repeated, supervised practice. The therapeutic philosophy underlying the treatments and the ability to adjust the treatments appropriately to individual patients can only be learned through close study of actual cases in a clinical setting under the tutelage of an experienced naturopathic hydrotherapist. The following description of the constitutional treatment is not meant as a substitute for either of these practical training experiences but rather as an introduction to those who will be receiving such clinical training and as a review and reference guide for those who have already received it.

DEFINITION:

a series of hot and cold compresses applied to the chest, abdomen and back in conjunction with mild sine wave or other electrical stimulation to the back and abdomen

MATERIALS:

2 blankets (more for a chilly patient or cool environment)
5 towels
oral thermometer
pillow
container(s) for urine specimens
refractometer
stethoscope
treatment table
sine wave machine or other apparatus with electrical source
prescription record sheet (see page 212)

PROCEDURE AND MECHANISM:

Phase	Position	Procedure	Duration	Mechanism
Preparation	supine	obtain urine specimen measure/record sp. gravity spread one blanket lengthwise on table with pillow at head have patient undress from waist up and lie down and cover self with blanket take/record oral temp test sine machine on self to make sure it works properly place warm, moist sine pads between patient's shoulder blades at the level of T_5 pull patient's lower garment down from waist to pelvis insert towel in waist to protect clothing auscultate heart and abdomen (see Chapter 28) palpate and percuss abdomen write prescription for treatment according to findings and conditions (see page 211)	5-8 min.	
#1	supine	prepare 2 towels as hot as possible, dry enough so they don't drip but wet enough so that a light wringing brings forth water expose patient's chest and abdomen test towels on your wrist and on patient to make sure they are not too hot apply towels one on top of the other over chest and abdomen from the clavicle to the pelvis, each folded in half (giving 4 layers total) cover patient with blanket	5 min.	short hot → dilation → ↑ circulation → ↑ metabolism both in skin and underlying organs

CONSTITUTIONAL APPROACH

Phase	Position	Procedure	Duration	Mechanism
Transition A	supine	prepare 1 cold towel just dry enough so that gentle wringing does not bring forth water prepare 1 hot towel as those in phase #1 open blanket and apply new hot towel on top of 2 original towels flip these 3 towels over on chest and abdomen, making sure new towel is not too hot remove original 2 towels, leaving the one new hot towel apply cold towel over top of single remaining hot towel inform patient that cold application is coming		short hot → as above also intensifies treatment by increasing contrast with following cold
#2	supine	flip these two towels over onto chest and abdomen remove new hot towel, leaving only cold towel close blanket cover chest and abdomen additionally with second blanket folded in quarters apply sine surge gradually to tolerance do not end this phase until towel is warm	10 min. or until towel is warm	short cold → constriction → dilation → ↑ circulation in skin and organs short cold →↑ wbc →↑ immunity →↑ rbc →↑ nutrition →↑ metabolism → detoxification sine wave → muscle contraction → ↑ metabolism ↑ circulation → sympathetic n.n. stim to abdom. organs, e.g., liver, pancreas and stomach also, absorption of non-ionized water from towel (¼ cup, according to Dr. Carroll) (see page 145)

CONSTITUTIONAL TREATMENT

Phase	Position	Procedure	Duration	Mechanism
Transition B	supine	turn off sine machine remove second blanket open first blanket remove towel place 1 sine pad at thora-columbar junction and 1 pad over solar plexus or other abdominal point as prescribed place shotbag or sandbag over abdominal pad to hold it in place replace first blanket as it was		
# 3	supine	apply sine surge to tolerance check on patient periodically to make sure sine wave is comfortable	10 min.	sine wave → muscle contraction →↑ metabolism →↑ circulation →↑ peristalsis → nervous stimulation to abdominal organs
Transition C	supine	turn off sine machine open blanket and remove electrical pads		
	prone	have patient turn onto stomach move protective waist towel from front to back cover with first wool blanket		
#4	prone	prepare two hot towels and apply to patient's back see phase #1 above	5 min.	same as phase #1 with added emphasis on spinal cord
Transition D	prone	prepare 1 cold and 1 hot towel put fresh hot towel over 2 original hot towels flip these 3 towels over and remove 2 original towels put cold towel over remaining towel		short hot increases contrast (see Transition A above)

Phase	Position	Procedure	Duration	Mechanism
#5	prone	flip these and remove hot towel, leaving only cold towel close blanket and cover back with 4 folds of second blanket after 10 minutes feel under blankets over upper spine to see if skin and towel are warm if warm, terminate treatment	10 min.	short cold (see Phase # 2 above) with added emphasis on spinal cord
		if not warm, give light stroking and percussion through all the blanket thicknesses	1 min.	stimulates vasodilation which warms skin
		wait 1-2 minutes then recheck for warmth repeat, as necessary, until warm do not terminate treatment until warm once warm, remove blankets and towel	1-2 min.	
Conclusion	prone	dry back very lightly with towel used to protect clothing		
		retake oral temperature and record (may start earlier if desired) rest patient as possible or necessary have patient dress obtain second urine specimen measure and record specific gravity record any significant patient reactions to the treatment	5-8 min.	

Note: The importance of never removing a cold towel before the patient has warmed it up cannot be overemphasized. If a cold phase is terminated before the patient's response to it is complete, the treatment will be ineffective, and it may chill the patient. If the patient subsequently catches cold, he or she may attribute it to the improperly applied treatment and discontinue the therapy.

VARIATIONS & OPTIONS:

If oral temperature is less than 97 ° F, warm the patient before the standard treatment (e.g., with a series of 2 hot towels for 3 minutes each pair or with hot packs) and then treat accordingly. Do not give the standard treatment to a patient whose oral temperature is less than 97 °F without first raising it.

If oral temperature is between 97-98 ° F, use an extra pair of hot towels during the first and fourth phases. Leave the first pair of hot towels on 4 minutes, then apply the second pair of hot towels for 2 minutes and proceed normally with the subsequent phases. This is referred to as "4/2" in hydrotherapeutic shorthand.

If oral temperature is between 98-99 ° F, give the standard treatment.

If oral temperature is between 99-100 ° F, shorten the first and fourth (i.e., the hot) phases from 5 to 3 minutes and lengthen the second and fifth (cold) phases from 10-15 minutes.

If oral temperature is between 100-101 ° F, shorten the first and fourth (hot) phases to 2 minutes and lengthen the second and fifth (cold) phases to 15 minutes.

If oral temperature is greater than 101 ° F, shorten the first and fourth (hot) phases to 1 minute and lengthen the second and fifth (cold) phases from 15-20 minutes.

If patient complains of feeling chilly, regardless of the temperature, give the "4/2" as described above for phases one and four.

If lung congestion is present, give the "4/2."

If the rheumatic diathesis (constitutional predisposition to painful musculoskeletal ailments and sensitivity to cold) is present, give the "4/2."

If extreme peripheral pain is present, place a hot compress over it during phase 1.

If significant congestion is present in any cavity (head, pelvis, chest, abdomen), heat should be applied to the feet, especially during the cold phases, and especially if the feet are already cold.

In cases of chronic pelvic problems (e.g., involving the ovaries, uterus, prostate or bladder) one of two options should be followed, if possible:

a. don't use the sine wave but apply instead 5 minutes of high frequency or short wave diathermy over the affected area during the third phase, or
b. give the standard treatment with 5 minutes of high frequency or short wave to the affected area at the end of the treatment.

Note: never switch electrical modalities, e.g., from sine to short wave, without an intervening set of hot and cold towels.

During a healing crisis (see Chapter 32) without fever, the order of the treatment should be changed according to one of the two following options:

phase 1: 5 min. hot to back
phase 2: 10 min. cold to back
phase 3: 10 min. interscapular sine wave ("5-5")
phase 4: 10 min. sine to abdomen and thoracolumbar junction
phase 5: 5 min. hot to chest/abdomen
phase 6: 10 min. cold to chest/abdomen

or . . .

phase 1: 5 min. hot to back
phase 2: 10 min. cold to back
phase 3: 10 min. sine to abdomen and thoracolumbar junction
phase 4: 5 min. hot to chest/abdomen
phase 5: 10 min. cold to chest/abdomen with interscapular sine wave ("5-5")

If patient is tense and anxious, apply one of the above healing crisis variations.

If the patient is overly stressed, for whatever reason, apply one of the above healing crisis variations.

For conditions involving local problems such as leg ulcers, fractures, headaches, and cellulitis, an extra phase of continuous or rapidly-pulsed sine wave may be applied to perception between what would normally be the third and fourth phases of the treatment with one pad over or distal to the involved area and the other over the spinal level governing innervation to the involved area., e.g., for an ulcer on the left leg of a diabetic patient, one sine pad would be placed distal to the ulcer and one pad over the left side of the lower lumbar spine. No localized treatment should be given until after five standard constitutional treatments have been administered.

In treating children (under five feet in height is a useful dividing point) no interscapular or "5-5" sine wave should be used in the second phase, and no additional hot towel for the transition flip from the hot to cold phases should be used. In addition, the length of the hot and cold phases in pediatric cases may be doubled, e.g., the first and fourth phases would be 10 minutes hot and the second and fifth phases would be 20 minutes cold. This last change of times, employed by Dr. Scott, is optional.

Note: All the times mentioned in these instructions, such as 5 minutes and "$4/2$," are approximate. Your clinical judgement is more important than blind adherence to rules and timetables.

INDICATIONS:

Because of its ability to improve the overall nutrition and boost the immunity, constitutional hydrotherapy may be useful in almost any condition; however, it has been found particularly suited to:

- digestive tract problems, such as
  - dyspepsia
  - Crohn's disease
  - irritable bowel syndrome
  - ulcerative colitis
- respiratory problems, such as
  - chronic asthma
  - bronchitis
  - pleurisy

- infectious diseases, such as
  - colds
  - flu
  - lymphangitis
- female reproductive problems, such as
  - premenstrual syndrome
  - dysmenorrhea
  - infertility
- immune deficiency problems, such as
  - cancer
  - environmental hypersensitivity
- circulatory problems, such as
  - varicose veins
  - hemorrhoids
  - Raynaud's disease
  - hypertension
- and other ailments, such as
  - arthritis
  - diabetes
  - depression
  - obesity
  - psoriasis

CONTRAINDICATIONS:

- acute bladder infection
- acute asthma
- malignant fever
- patient with oral temperature less than 97° F
- fear of treatment
- standard contraindications for sine wave applications, e.g., over a menstruating or gravid uterus or over malignancy or blood clot, should be observed (see Chapter 29)
- likewise, standard contraindications for short wave diathermy and high frequency should be observed if these modalities are included in the treatment (see Chapter 29)

Note: Dr. Leo Scott confirms O. G. Carroll's claim that the water absorbed by the patient from the cold towels plays an important role in the effectiveness of the constitutional treatment. In Dr. Scott's own words:

> I made a study at the time of weighing both the hot and cold packs before and after application on hundreds of patients using a gram scale. The hot packs varied little before and after application. The cold packs invariably weighed less, even though the skin was dry. The more water that was absorbed the faster the improvement. Those who absorbed the most got well the fastest. If there was any secret to Dr. Carroll's tremendous success it was this principle and the timing of the applications as based on the patient's temperature.

Dr. Carroll believed this water was non-ionized and that, therefore, it had special qualities as a toxin solvent.

We strongly recommend that students or doctors interested in incorporating Dr. Carroll's constitutional treatment into their practices review Dr. Harold Dick's videotapes at the NCNM library and preceptor one week or more with Drs. Dick and Scott in Spokane, Washington.

28. AUSCULTATION

Traditionally in constitutional hydrotherapy auscultation of the chest and abdomen has been one of the most important bases for individualizing the treatments, not just from patient-to-patient, but from day-to-day in the same patient. Drs. Carroll, Dick, Scott and Bastyr each evolved their own personal methods for understanding the heart and bowel sounds, but they are all based, more or less, on the teachings of Russell Trall. (Dr. Scott also recommends Loewenberg's *Medical Diagnosis.*) The subjective nature of some of the characterizations of the heart sounds makes them difficult to teach. We can only introduce you to the general concepts and encourage those of you who are interested to pursue studies with Drs. Dick, Scott and Bastyr. Those with a background in Chinese pulse diagnosis may have a better feel for this type of approach.

The heart is auscultated over the apex or the PMI (point of maximum impulse). Dr. Carroll preferred a large auscultory bell with rubber from a latex exam glove stretched over it for a diaphragm. He found this not only transmitted the sounds but also the pressure which can be felt in the auditory canals. However, a standard stethoscope may be used. The heart sounds are listened to for rate, rhythm and quality.

A fast rate over 82 beats per minute may suggest stress, toxicity, fever, anxiety or a hyperthyroid condition. A slow rate of less than 60 beats per minute may suggest a bowel, gallbladder or liver problem, or a conditioned athlete.

In general, arrhythmias suggest digestive difficulties, which makes sense when you remember that many myocardial infarctions occur after large meals. Specifically, skipped beats are associated with problems of the lower stomach (the pylorus) and extra beats are associated with upper stomach problems as, for example, when a meal is taken which does not digest. Other irregularities of the rhythm may indicate a heart muscle problem resulting from general toxicity.

The quality of the heart beat is the most significant factor, and its wide array of possibilities makes it the most difficult as well. In general, the most important distinction to make is whether or not the heart is straining to push the blood. In the words of Dr. Dick, if it sounds like a diesel truck going uphill, then it is straining, which means there is toxicity, and you have a problem. If it sounds like a diesel running downhill or on a flat stretch, then the heart is not straining, the toxicity is diminished, and clinically you are going in the right direction.

Beyond that there are other useful distinctions which may be made. Sharp sounds mean irritation. This is commonly found in acute cases and is frequently associated with increased bowel sounds. Full, mushy sounds signify congestion. This is more commonly found in chronic cases and is usually associated with decreased bowel sounds. Hard, bounding sounds are regarded as a combination of irritation and congestion. Small sounds suggest weakness. In general the quality of the first sound is associated with organs above the diaphragm while the second sound is associated with organs below the diaphragm.

Further, specific organ involvement may be deduced by the following:

- a watch-like "tick-tock" quality of the sounds with no pause between the cycles, like water dripping, suggests a liver problem;
- a similar ticking quality but with a pause between cycles suggests small intestine involvement;
- an elongated second sound means a large intestine problem; if the elongated S_2 has a wiry quality, the descending colon is involved; if it has a full quality, the ascending colon is implicated;
- when S_2 is not only elongated but also hard, full and wiry, uterine problems are suspected;

when S_2 is feathery, i.e., when it fades gradually, the bladder is involved;

heart sounds with a pecking quality suggest difficulties with the spleen;

wiry, vibrating sounds suggest stomach irritation;

heavy, thudding sounds, like a rock falling, suggest the kidney;

metallic, ringing qualities of the sounds call the heart itself into question.

In addition to the heart, the abdomen is also examined. Observation is the first step. If a strong celiac pulse, which signifies toxicity, is present, it is often visible in the area of the solar plexus.In thin patients spasms of the intestines and the abdominal muscles may occasionally be observed. Auscultation over all segments of the abdomen is next (see Figure 7).

FIGURE 7
(DIVISIONS OF THE ABDOMEN)

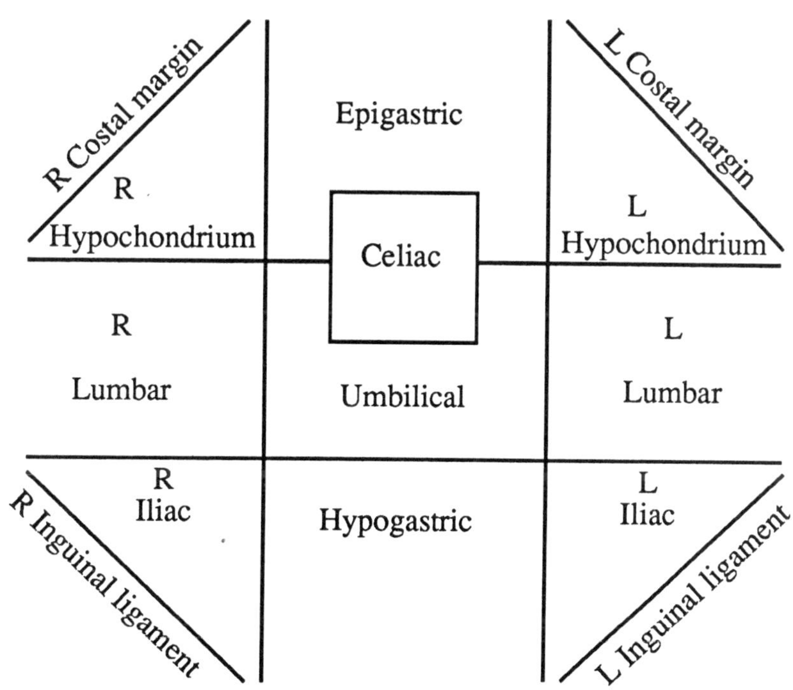

If bowel sounds are absent over any area, listen for a longer time or come back to that spot later and check again. If sounds are still absent, congestion is present. The area should then be palpated. If tender, spasm is probably present and proximal impaction should be ruled out. If bowel sounds are increased and have a high-pitched quality, like elephants trumpeting, these are borborygmi and suggest bowel irritation such as would be found in Crohn's disease, ulcerative colitis or irritable bowel syndrome. The celiac pulse may also be auscultated and palpated. Again, the celiac pulse is a keynote of toxicity.

The importance of these examinations is that they guide the practitioner to proper adjustments of the constitutional treatments. There is a good correlation between the heart and abdominal exams. The problem area suggested by the heart sounds is confirmed or not by the findings of the abdominal exam. In practical terms, these exams tell us where or where not to put the sine wave pads during the normal third phase of the constitutional treatment. The meaning of these correlative findings is summarized in the following chart (Figure 8).

FIGURE 8
HEART SOUNDS

Quality	Significance	Bowel Correlation	3rd Phase Change
Sharp	acute irritation	increased bowel sounds	high frequency
Full, mushy	chronic congestion	decreased bowel sounds	diathermy
hard, bounding	irritation + congestion	celiac pulse	sine/celiac
Small tick-tock w/o pause	general weakness liver involvement	right-sided findings	sine/R hypochondrium
Small tick-tock w/pause	small intestine	central findings	sine/umbilicus
Increased S_1	above diaphragm	normal bowel sounds	
Increased S_2	below diaphragm	absent, normal or abnormal sounds	sine or h.f. as indicated
Long S_2	large intestine	epigastric findings	sine/epigastrium
Long, wiry S_2	descending colon	left-sided findings	sine/L Lumbar
Long, full S_2	ascending colon	right-sided findings	sine/R Lumbar
Long, full, wiry, hard S_2	uterus/prostate	normal bowel sounds	h.f./hypogastrium
Feathery S_2	bladder	normal bowel sounds	
Pecking	spleen	normal bowel sounds	
heavy, thudding	kidney	normal bowel sounds	
metallic, ringing	heart	normal bowel sounds	

The foregoing chartings are guidelines. Common sense must be used. Occasionally there may be two or three major organ findings, in which case the 3rd phase modality can be distributed clockwise in 3-5 minute segments to the various areas. For example, in a patient with findings throughout the large intestine, sine wave could be applied three minutes over the right lumbar region, 3 minutes over the epigastrium and 3 minutes over the left lumbar area.

Of course, all exam findings are more valuable if compared before and after treatment.

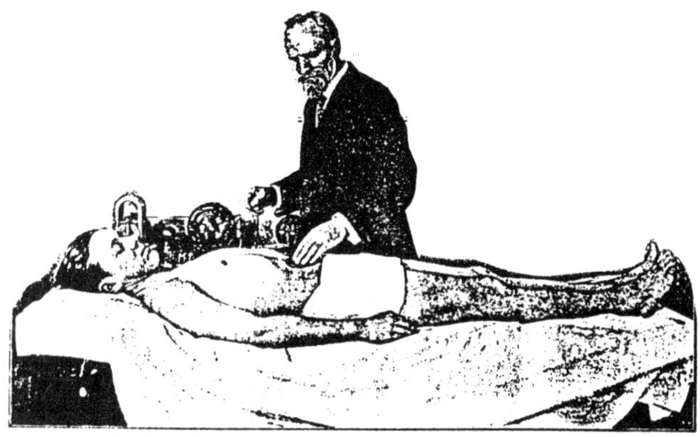

29. HYDROTHERAPY AND ELECTROTHERAPY

Electrotherapy and hydrotherapy are similar treatments in that both work through the skin and nerves with direct local and indirect reflex effects on the circulation of blood and lymph. When combined, these modalities are not only compatible but also synergistic. The increased vascularity of tissue treated with hot and cold water applications increases the electrical conductivity of that tissue as does the external moisture from the water treatments. The muscle contractions caused by sine wave application in the constitutional treatment add a mechanical component to the thermic impressions of the hot and cold applications which enhance the circulatory effects.

There are four basic electrical modes used with hydrotherapy — sine wave, diathermy (short wave), galvanic and high frequency. We are speaking of them here primarily as third-phase components in the constitutional treatment. It should be noted that if diathermy, galvanic or high frequency are used in the third phase of the constitutional treatment, sine wave would *not* be administered to the T_5 area during the second phase. Remember the already-stated rule: do not switch electrical modes without an intervening set of hot and cold towels. This is to avoid overstimulation.

How do you know which form of electricity to employ in your constitutional treatments? Let's discuss this question.

Sine wave is the standard "all-purpose" electrical mode, the optimal frequency being 12-18 h_z, the best surge rate being 8-12/minute. We have already discussed the rationale for its use during the demonstration of the constitutional treatment (see page 138). Before going over when and when not to use it, let's take a minute to elaborate on its salutory effects. Some people think it is some sort of hocus-pocus — you put electricity over something and it helps, like kissing it and making it better. But listen to the words of Kellogg:

> The application of the sinusoidal current to the abdomen alone is sufficient to produce great relief in a large class of neurasthenics . . . the pathological foundation of neurasthenia (in many cases) is unquestionably located in the abdominal region and consists in a disturbance of the sympathetics growing out of the passive congestion or stagnation of the portal circulation . . . Permanent relief is obtained only by development of the abdominal muscles, thus restoring the intra-abdominal tension which, by compression of the portal vessels and the viscera, relieves them of their surplus blood, and thus relieves the irritation of the sympathetic centers which produce depression, insomnia, irritability, backache, headache, and the infinite variety of distressing symptoms known only to neurasthenics . . . By the application of the slow sinusoidal current to the abdomen vigorous intermittent contraction of the abdomen muscles may be produced, and, as a result, their tone may be increased so that through compression of the abdominal veins the stagnated blood is pushed along; the half-asphyxiated viscera are cleared of their toxin-laden blood; the sympathetic centers receive a fresh, invigorating blood supply; the diaphragm is strengthened, and hence the breathing is reinforced and the blood better aerated; the heart's action becomes more energetic, metabolism is encouraged, and every vital process is improved.

Sine wave may be routinely employed as part of the constitutional treatment. It is especially indicated when a celiac pulse (see page 149) is present. However, there are important exceptions to its use, especially in women. Sine wave should not be used over a menstruating uterus, especially if pain is present; in such a case high frequency should be employed. Likewise, in mastitis, high frequency would be appropriate over the involved breast tissue but not sine wave. In conditions affecting the bladder, uterus and ovaries, sine wave should not be applied directly over these organs; high frequency or short wave diathermy should be substituted and may be alternated every other treatment. In chronic gastrointestinal tract problems where no peristalsis is present (as determined by the absence of bowel sounds on auscultation), diathermy is the electrical modality of choice.

This is not the place to review the proper use of *short wave diathermy*. Please consult your electrotherapy texts for that. As suggested above, its use in the constitutional treatment is indicated in problems affecting the pelvic and abdominal viscera, especially if peristalsis is diminished or absent. Important contraindications would be fever, local bleeding, (e.g., ulcer, colitis, menstruation) and acutely inflamed viscus. In these cases high frequency would be used in its place. In treatments over the pelvis, remember to have the patient empty his or her bladder first. Also remember to use a half inch of dry towel or felt pad between the short wave applicator and the skin.

Galvanism may also be integrated into the constitutional treatment. Positive galvanism is used primarily against inflammatory swelling, because of its ability to constrict vessels and shrink tissue, and negative galvanism is used against fibrosis, because of its ability to cause tissue dilation. Please refer to a good physiotherapy text for a properly detailed explanation of the uses of galvanism.

You may be least familiar with the high frequency apparatus. High frequency is basically static electricity generated into a glass tube which is applied to the skin overlying the affected areas. It is called for in cases of *acute inflammatin and congestion with severe pain and/or fever*. It is good in cases of fever because it neither adds nor generates heat. Some practitioners call it the *"Belladonna of electricity."* (Remember, sharpness in the heart sounds suggests inflammation, and fullness indicates congestion; see page 148). Acute appendicitis and kidney abscess would be examples in this category. Another indication is in *respiratory ailments, like pneumonia and bronchitis, in babies and children*. Finally, it can be used in chronic cases to help regenerate damaged organs and tissue, e.g., in diabetic skin ulcers and kidney failure.

We will now give a brief demonstration of the high frequency unit. When you turn on the generator, you notice a crackling sound and see the dancing violet light it produces. Cornstarch should be used over the treatment area to absorb moisture. Start with the applicator on your hand so you can properly judge intensity, then transfer the applicator to the treatment area. This avoids sparking as the current jumps from the applicator to the skin which can be painful and/or frightening. Keep the instrument head moving over the treatment area *in constant contact with the skin* for about 5 minutes. If there are two areas, use 4 minutes on the more important area and 2 minutes on the other. For very small areas use shorter time periods. At the end of the treatment turn the machine off before removing the applicator, or transfer the applicator back to your hand, again, to avoid sparking.

When you think of high frequency, think of *soothing* for the pain of inflammation and congestion.

The most effective high frequency unit is the Vita-Ray from the Edgar Cayce Foundation. This unit combines the high frequency with positive and negative galvanism. A big problem with high frequency is that it can disturb radio waves. The Federal Communications Commission has gone after high frequency users for that reason. Operating the high frequency in a "Cage of Faraday" might help mitigate this problem. The Via-Ray supposedly cannot be sold or transported across state borders, but, theoretically, it can be built and used within the same state. See your attorney about these questions.

A simple unit which makes only high frequency is available from Arrow Glass Co., 710 Vandustrial Drive, Westmont, IL 60559. Ask for the #411 Generator Case which comes with the #1 General Electrode. At last notice the cost was about $120.00. It is sold as an electrolysis unit for hair removal and is not so powerful as the Vita-Ray; however, it is a viable option.

Remember, in applying high frequency, to *avoid moisture and avoid metal.*

30. HYDROTHERAPY AND BOTANICAL MEDICINE

You have all had extensive courses in botanical medicine. What we plan to give you here is a brief summary of how Dr. Carroll, who was an accomplished botanist, used herbs in conjunction with hydrotherapy. Dr. O. G. Carroll knew literally thousands of herbs, but he kept all his therapeutic formulas simple. He believed that each herb was a complex medicine compounded by nature and, therefore, that it was unnecessary to mix a lot of herbs together in a fancy botanical formula. Almost all the herbs he employed were gastrointestinal tract tonics, which improve digestion, and laxatives, which promote detoxification. Even the nervines he used, such as skullcap and valerian, influence the bowel.

Dr. Carroll used herbs as encapsulated powders, tinctures, teas and salves. The following are his most important capsule formulas as used by Dr. Harold Dick.

"C" Capsules:

2 parts (by weight) Wormwood (*Artemisia absinthium*)
1 part Gentian (*Gentiana lutea*)
1 part Cape Aloes (*Aloes socotrina*)

"C" Capsules are a combination of digestive aid and laxative. The wormwood is tonic to the upper G.I. tract. The gentian stimulates the production of HCl. The powdered gum of cape aloes is tonic to the lower G.I. tract. The usual adult recommendation is one "00" capsule per day in warm water.

"50" Capsules:

2 parts Gentian *(Gentiana lutea)*
1 part Skullcap *(Scutellaria lateriflora)*

"50" Capsules are used in cases of poor digestion related to stress. The gentian improves the appetite and digestion by increasing HCl production in the stomach. The skullcap calms the nerves and beneficially influences the G.I. tract, especially the stomach, via the nervous system. One "00" capsule in warm water for flatulence.

"G" Capsules (also called "Special G"):

Gentian only (*Gentiana lutea*)

"G" Capsules are indicated in cases of indigestion, especially when the saliva is found to be acidic. As mentioned, gentian increases HCl secretion which starts the digestive process. One "00" capsule in warm water before meals for up to ten days. Do not use if nausea is present.

"Nervine" Capsules:

1 part Skullcap (*Scutellaria lateriflora*)
1 part Valerian (*Valeriana officinalis*)

"Nervine" Capsules calm the nerves. Skullcap is a central nervous system calmative with indirect effects on the G.I. tract. Valerian is a C.N.S. calmative with direct tonic effects upon the digestive system. One "00" capsule with meals. May also be used at bedtime for insomnia.

"WW" Capsules:

Wormwood only (*Artemisia absinthium)*

"WW" Capsules are indicated in digestive problems involving the upper G.I. tract, because wormwood stimulates the production and secretion of bile and gastric juices. They are also used in asthma and other mucous conditions (one "00" capsule before bed) because of wormwood's ability to liquify mucus.

"42" Capsules:

2 parts Wormwood (*Artemisia absinthium*)
1 part Cape Aloes (*Aloes socotrina*)

"42" Capsules are the most commonly used of Dr. Carroll's capsules. They are indicated for everything from constipation, atonic dyspepsia, round worms and pinworms to colds, angina, asthma, etc. The wormwood works on the upper G.I. tract to improve digestion while the cape aloes is a slow large intestine purgative which empties the bowel in 10-15 hours. One "00" capsule per day offers strong laxative action, or, in pressing cases, two capsules may be taken every four hours until the bowels move. The "42" Cocktail is indicated in acute conditions with pain and irritation such as angina and asthma. A "42" Cocktail consists of two "42" Capsules emptied into a glass, mixed with one ounce of warm water and drunk. This is followed by a chaser of more water to clean out remnants of the herbs from the glass and wash the bitter taste from the mouth. The next meal should be skipped. The "42" Cocktail acts rapidly, in 5-10 minutes to "sweeten the stomach" and relieve pain. The Bible says, bitter in the mouth, sweet in the stomach, and, as Dr. Dick says, "God knows it's bitter." Colds may be aborted if a "42" Cocktail is taken at the first sign and the next one to two meals are skipped. Dr. Dick gives all his patients a supply of "42's" to keep at home so that he can prescribe a "cocktail" over the phone when necessary. Do not give for nausea unless due to food poisoning.

The following are a number of the herbal tea formulas used by Dr. Carroll and his followers. Many are based on the recipes of Father Kneipp. General directions for use would be: place two tablespoons of cut and sifted herb in 1½ cups of boiling water; stir and let steep for at least 10 minutes; then strain and drink.

"Kidney" Formula:

2 parts Marjoram
1 part Elder (*Sambucus canadensis*)

This is a diuretic formula to be used in cases of edema. Elder, a strong diuretic and alterative, is the active ingredient. The marjoram has a soothing action on the renal tissue.

"Enuresis" Formula:

2 parts St. Johnswort (*Hypericum*)
1 part Dwarf Elder (*Aralia*)

This combination helps control excessive urination.

"Edema" Formula:

2 parts Motherwort (*Leonorus cardiaca)*
2 parts Dwarf Elder (*Aralia*)
1 part Buchu (optional)

This is used similarly to the "Kidney" Formula, especially with cardiac involvement.

"Hemorrhage" Formula:

2 parts Amaranthus (or *Bayberry bark* if Amaranthus is unavailable)
1 part Rush (*Equisetum arvense*)

General formula for hemorrhage, e.g., bleeding piles.

"Uterine Hemorrhage" Formula:

2 parts Amaranthus (or *Bayberry bark*)
1 part Leopard's Bane (*Arnica*) (potentially toxic in high doses)

For uterine bleeding, e.g., postpartum.

"Bowel Hemorrhage" Formula:

1 part Amaranthus (or *Bayberry bark*)
1 part Rush (*Equisetum arvense*)

"Amenorrhea" Formula:

2 parts Uva Ursi *(Arctostaphylos)*
1 part Dwarf Elder (Aralia)

For a late or suppressed period.

"Dysmenorrhea" Formula:

2 parts Squaw Vine (*Mitchella*)
1 part Leopard's Bane (*Arnica*) (potentially toxic in high doses)

For pain during the menstrual period.

"Pregnancy" Formula:

1 part Marjoram
1 part Squaw Vine (*Mitchella*)

"Menstrual Regulation" Formula:

3 parts Leopard's Bane (*Arnica*) (potentially toxic in high doses)
3 parts Squaw Vine (*Mitchella*)
2 parts Rush (*Equisetum arvense*)

To regulate a too great or too little flow.

"Bladder" Formula:

1 part Rush (*Equisetum arvense*)
1 part Squaw Vine (*Mitchella*)
1 part Marjoram

For inflammation and infection of the bladder.

"Hot Flash" Formula:

2 parts Uva Ursi *(Arctostaphylos)*
1 part Shepherd's Purse (*Capsella*)

For hot flashes and other menopausal symptoms.

"Varicose Vein" Formula:

2 parts Stone Root (*Collinsonia*)
2 parts Oregon Grape (*Berberis*)
1 part Witch hazel (*Hamamelis*)

For varicosities including hemorrhoids, internal and external.

In terms of alcoholic extracts the following formulas were used by Dr. Carroll:

"Liver" Formula:

2 parts *Chionanthus* ∅(*tincture*)
2 parts *Chelidonium* ∅
1 part *Podophyllum* ∅(contraindicated in pregnancy)

10 drops in a half glass of water 2-3 times per day for sluggish hepatic function.

"Heart Drops" Formula:

2 parts *Cretagus* ∅
1 part Cactus ∅

10 drops of the above mixture in a glass of water twice daily for cardiac infirmity.

The following, more complex, formulas for making larger quantities for storage are also given:

"Blood Tonic":

1 cup Pipsissewa (dry cut)
1 cup *Echinacea*
½ cup Gentian
½ cup *Podophyllum* (contraindicated in pregnancy)

Add above dry herbs to 11 pints of water and boil well for 5-10 minutes. Strain, bottle and keep refrigerated. Add oil of wintergreen to taste. Take 1 tablespoon 3 times per day.

"Cough Syrup":

4 tablespoons Rhubarb root
2 cups honey
2 cups hot water
2 teaspoons *Capsicum* ∅
2 tablespoons essence of Peppermint
2 tablespoons baking soda

Mix rhubarb root and soda together, then add honey to make a paste. Add hot water and stir until all is dissolved. Add *Capsicum* and peppermint last. Bottle. Give in small quantities — the tip of a teaspoon — as needed.

"Brown" or "Healing" Salve:

½ tablet Argyrol (for color)
½ tablespoon Tannic acid
¼ tablespoon Zinc oxide
½ tablespoon Turmeric
Witch hazel extract sufficient to make a paste
1 pound vaseline (or honey)

Mix , tannic acid, zinc oxide and turmeric. Add enough witch hazel to make a paste. Mix and then add vaseline (or honey). Dissolve argyrol in 1½ teaspoons of water and mix it into the compound. Stir well and store in small containers.

To use: apply sparingly to a thin piece of wet cotton cloth or several layers of gauze. Place over injury and cover with wool (except for sunburn). Leave on until dry.
The brown salve is used in treating sunburn, bruises, alkali burns, sprains and non-infected cuts.

"Black" or "Drawing" Salve:

1 heaping tablespoon cut Echinacea
1 heaping tablespoon cut White Oak bark
1 heaping tablespoon cut Pipsissewa
1 cup water
⅔ tablespoon Gallic acid
Witch hazel extract sufficient to dissolve Gallic acid
2 oz. Ichthyol
2 pounds vaseline

Place herbs in 1 cup of water and bring to a boil. Allow to boil for 10 minutes, then cool and strain. Mix gallic acid with just enough witch hazel to dissolve it. To this solution add ⅓ cup of tea strained from the above herbs. Add ichthyol and vaseline and mix thoroughly. Store in several small containers.

To use: apply sparingly to a small, wet cotton cloth or several layers of moistened gauze. Place over affected area, cover with wool and leave on until dry. The black salve is used on infections, boils, stings, puncture wounds and other septic injuries. It has a reputation for drawing out fluid, pus and tumors. Once the black salve has eliminated the inflammation/infection, then the brown salve should be used in its place.

"White" or "Itch" Salve:

3 tablespoons cornstarch
1 tablespoon Zinc oxide
Witch hazel extract sufficient to make a paste
1 pound vaseline

Mix cornstarch and zinc oxide. Stir in just enough witch hazel to make a paste. Mix thoroughly with vaseline and store in small containers.

To use: apply sparingly to affected parts and cover with a light, dry cloth. White salve is used to sooth eczema and other skin rashes. It is also used for burns from a stove or iron and for acid burns.

There is much more which could be said about herbs as used by Dr. Carroll and his followers. For example, Dr. Leo Scott's booklet, "You Can Help Yourself To Health," explains the use of herbs according to the Physio-medicalist system, a vitalistic approach to botanical medicine which rejects those herbs with potentially toxic properties. The following categories of herbs, as presented by Dr. Scott, suggest some of their uses.

Generals:

Tonics: *Hydrastis, Gentiana, Populus, Berberis*
Stimulants: *Capsicum, Zingiber, Mentha*
Nervines: *Valeriana, Scutellaria*

Specifics:

Alteratives: *Echinacea, Arctium, Chimaphila*
Anthelmintics: *Artemisia, Dryopteris*
Astringents: *Hamamelis, Myrica*
Demulcents: *Symphytum, Marrubium, Althea*
Diaphoretics: *Achillea, Asclepias, Eupatorium perfoliatum*
Diuretics: *Arctostaphylos, Barosma, Eupatorium purpureum, Leonurus*
Pelvics: *Arctostaphylos, Capsella, Viburnum, Dioscorea*

For a thoroughgoing explanation of the naturopathic uses of these and other herbs please consult *Herbal Medication, A Clinical and Dispensatory Handbook* by A. W. Priest and L.R. Priest (London, L.N. Fowler and Co., Ltd., 1982).

Of course, Dr. Carroll's and Dr. Scott's herbs are not the only ones compatible with hydrotherapy, nor are all herbs which are compatible with hydrotherapy used internally. Father Kneipp and his followers frequently added herbs to the various baths they administered, e.g., valerian for nervous conditions, horsetail for bladder problems, oak bark for skin conditions and thyme for bacterial infections. Dr. Bluggermann's *Kneipp Vademecum* is a good source for these herbal baths. In addition, "Herbal Hydrotherapeutics," a paper on file at the National College of Naturopathic Medicine library by Drs. Gloria Schwartz and Joe Coletto, has excellent recipes, especially for eye baths.

We should conclude with Dr. Dick's admonition not to overdo the herbs. He feels herbs are to provide temporary relief but not to cure. The cure comes later through the hydrotherapy. If you give the herbs for more than temporary relief, a homeopathic proving may occur and complicate matters. In his words, "True cure is incompatible with maintenance therapy."

31. HYDROTHERAPY AND NUTRITION

"Our head cook is our chief pharmacist."

— Henry Lindlahr

Hydrotherapy has a synergistic relationship with all other natural therapies but none more so than with nutrition. If one of the most important functions of constitutional hydrotherapy is to detoxify the body, then one of the most important functions of healthful nutrition is to prevent intoxication. In our treatment protocols when we say, "remove the injurious foods," we mean to remove the foods which cause intoxication of the body. In general, this may be done by following these recommendations:

1) eat a diet rich in fresh, well-grown, well-prepared whole foods which are low in total calories, total fat, refined carbohydrates, food additives and stimulants;
2) orient the diet according to the person's blood type as per Dr. James D'Adamo's book, *One Man's Food Is . . . Someone Else's Poison,* i.e., a high protein diet for people with type O blood, a low protein diet for people with type A and a moderate protein diet for people with type B blood;
3) eliminate the foods to which the patient is intolerant or allergic.

There are numerous methods for determining food allergies — the elimination diet, challenge diet, Coca Pulse test, cytotoxic test, RAST test, skin test, sublingual test and others. None of these is entirely satisfactory. Today we will talk about the food intolerance method used by Dr. Carroll and his followers. It is not perfect either, but we will discuss the diets based on it because of the good clinical results they yield and because it is the method which has been used most extensively in conjunction with hydrotherapy.

Dr. Carroll practiced in Spokane, Washington from 1908 to 1963. During the 1930's he had a number of difficult cases which he could not cure. His auscultory exam (see Chapter 28) showed him that the problem in such cases was usually in the stomach. This was at a time when the concept of food allergy was almost unheard of, but Dr. Carroll experimented with different foods to find which were causing the problems. From these findings he was able to devise a method for identifying a patient's intolerance to a food, food group or combinations of foods which should be avoided because they cannot be digested and/or assimilated properly by that patient. Such an intolerance appears to be constitutional and unchanging, similar to one's blood type.

In the words of Dr. Carroll, "Health must at all times come from and be maintained by digested foods." When a person eats foods to which he is intolerant, these foods are not properly digested and assimilated. If these foods are high in carbohydrates, fermentation occurs; if they are high in proteins, putrification occurs. Both lead to a slow poisoning of the intestinal tract and eventually of all the body systems. Of course, each individual will respond differently to eating his food intolerance, depending on his constitutional strength. A person with a weak constitution is more susceptible to developing early symptoms of toxemia such as intestinal discomfort, skin eruptions, asthma, fatigue or mental confusion with ingestion of even minute amounts of the irritating food. Another person, with a strong constitution may eat his or her food intolerance several times a day without the slightest noticeable discomfort. However, it was Dr. Carroll's hypothesis, based on over 60 years of clinical observation, that even though a person's constitution was strong, if he ate his food intolerance, a strain was placed on the whole organism, and sooner or later systemic damage would occur. One is reminded that a tumor of the colon takes about 20 years to develop before the person experiences any symptoms. Similarly, a tumor of the breast takes about 12 years of development before it becomes palpable. During these years, the person may have felt great. *Prevention is always better than a cure.*

Some of Dr. Carroll's patients had their newborn babies evaluated before they could eat their food intolerance. These children generally developed remarkably well; they were intellectually sharp, emotionally stable and physically well-proportioned. An 82-year-old farmer of Umatilla, Oregon, was met recently at Dr. Leo Scott's clinic in Spokane. He said that forty years previously he could not walk from his house to his tractor without getting out of breath. At this time he had diabetes, hypertension and heart failure. His doctor had told him to sell his farm and to stay in bed, as he had less than six months to live. He then went to see Dr. Carroll in Spokane where he received hydrotherapy and was taken off his food intolerance which turned out to be dairy. He recovered rapidly and went back to farming. Afterward, he had his wife and children evaluated for their food intolerances and, through the years, also his grandchildren. He said that in forty years neither himself, his wife, children nor grandchildren has ever been sick. Moreover, he feels better at 82 than he did at 40. Again, *prevention is better than a cure.* Similar stories could be told by numerous other patients of Drs. Carroll, Dick or Scott. Please see "A New Lease On Life," by Beth Adele Beller.

It is commonly observed that the sick usually crave their food intolerances. Although, when elderly but healthy relatives of a sick patient have their diets checked for preventive purposes, it has often been found that they rarely ate the food which was determined to be their intolerance. Similarly, healthy children who are routinely evaluated for preventive purposes usually dislike their food intolerance, while the sick ones usually crave their food intolerances. As with an addictive drug, it seems that, at first, the person has a natural repulsion to his or her food intolerance, but if the use is further encouraged, he or she becomes addicted to it. Dr. Carroll used to say that the sick person craves his food intolerance because it feeds his disease process.

The major food groups for the intolerance are as follows:

1) *Dairy Group* (about 20% of those tested)
This includes all milks, cheeses, wheys, yogurts, and butters from any animal and any foods in which they are ingredients. Food additives such as sodium caseinate and lactic acid are milk derivatives. Some margarines have whey added to them. Soy milk is a good substitute. People with dairy intolerance who eat dairy products are susceptible to gastrointestinal problems such as Crohn's disease and ulcerative colitis, as well as asthma, sinusitis and mental dullness. About 70% of colitis patients are dairy reactive. The ailments resulting from dairy intolerance tend to manifest early in life.
2) *Fruit Group* (about 20% of those tested)
This includes all fruits, raw, cooked or dried; all berries, citrus and colas; all products made from fruits such as wine, vinegar, liquor, essential oil, or other fruit extract. Acerola berries, cranberries, coconut, olives, papaya, avocado, banana, and cheyote squash are considered fruits. Citric acid and citrus bioflavinoids are fruit derivatives. The following are *not* considered fruits: cantaloupe, watermelon, crenshaw, honey dew, muskmelon, casaba, ground cherries, rhubarb and tomatoes. People who eat their fruit intolerance are prone to arthritis, hypertension, autoimmune diseases and emotional problems.
3) *Eggs* (about 15% of those tested)
This includes all parts (whites, yolk and shell) of all poultry eggs and products containing them. Most pastries, ice creams, macaroni, spaghetti, candies, chewing gums and mayonnaise contain eggs. Commercial lecithin is usually from eggs (soy bean lecithin should be substituted). Beware of supplements with egg shell calcium. Patients who eat their egg intolerance tend toward headaches, skin problems and infections.
4) *Potatoes* (about 15% of those tested)
This includes white potatoes, sweet potatoes and yams and any foods containing potato products such as potato starch, modified starch, potato flour and potato water. Many prepared soups, noodles and sauces have such ingredients. Dextrose, a common

food additive, is frequently made from potato. Bread yeast, brewer's yeasts and nutritional yeasts are commonly grown on potato products. Potato intolerant patients tend toward the "rheumatic diathesis."

5) *Mine salt* (about 15% of those tested)
   This includes salt mined out of the earth and the many processed food products which contain it. People intolerant to mine salt are prone to gastrointestinal syndromes similar to those with dairy intolerance; in fact, the dairy and mine salt intolerance are often seen to coexist. Those intolerant to mine salt can also develop fatigue and headaches. Such people are rarely sensitive to sea salt which is, therefore, a good substitute.
6) *Meat* (about 10% of those tested)
   This includes beef, pork, mutton, venison and fowl, as well as meat products and by-products such as lard, gravy, jello, gelatin, marshmallows, some solid shortenings and margarines, and soups made from meat stock. Fish and sea food are *not* classified as meat. Sole, smelt and red snapper are recommended. Meat intolerances usually manifest themselves later in life in association with severe diseases such as multiple sclerosis and cancer.
7) *Fish* (less than 1% of those tested)
   Fish intolerance is rare and is found most frequently in patients of Asiatic heritage.
8) *Soy* (less than 1%)
   Soy intolerance likewise is rare and is found more often in Asiatics.
9) *Sugar* (about 20% of those tested)
   This includes cane or beet sugar regardless of whether it is white, brown or raw, as well as molasses, Karo and sorghum. Many prepared foods, including chewing gums, contain sugar. Read labels for dextrin, corn syrup solids, caramel, etc. Honey and pure maple syrup are not classified as sugar. Sugar intolerance manifests early and is therefore a big part of your pediatric practice. Middle ear and upper respiratory infections are common.

You can see that the frequency percentages add up to more than 100% which means that in some instances more than one basic intolerance may coexist in the same person.

In addition to these primary intolerances many people also have a combination intolerance. Most commonly these occur between cereal products and one of the other food groups, e.g.,

cereal products with dairy
cereal products with potatoes
cereal products with eggs
cereal products with fruits
cereal products with sugar.

By cereal products we mean all grains such as wheat, oats, cornmeal, corn-on-the-cob, rye, barley, flax, rice, wild rice, sesame, popcorn and millet, as well as all grain flours and everything made from them. Also included would be bran, wheat germ, cornstarch, hominy, grain liquor, malt vinegar, noodles, etc. Tapioca, soybean, arrowroot and buckwheat are not considered cereals. Flours and powders made from them may be used for baking.

In addition to the combination intolerances involving cereal there are three other combination intolerances:

meat with potatoes
meat with mine salt
and fruit with sugar.

The combination intolerance means that the foods involved are allowed but not within eight hours of each other.

Most patients are found to have a primary food intolerance, such as fruit, and then a secondary combination intolerance, such as meat and potatoes. This means that such a patient should not have fruit in any form at any time, but that he or she may have meat so long as it is not taken within eight hours of potatoes, and that he or she may have potatoes so long as they are not taken within eight hours of meat.

This is *not* the only useful system of nutrition which works well with hydrotherapy. Any method which accurately and reliably helps identify foods to which a patient may be allergic or intolerant is acceptable. We introduced you to this system because historically it was so closely identified with Dr. O. G. Carroll's use of constitutional hydrotherapy and because it is based on the very important principle of eliminating foods which, for whatever reason, have a toxic effect on a given patient. If you have another method for doing this which yields good results, then, by all means, employ it along with your hydrotherapy.

Due to limited time we have not gone into the food intolerance test procedures which, in any case, are beyond the scope of this course. Those interested in more information should consult Dr. Bill Carroll or Dr. Dick.

32. HEALING CRISIS

> "The effort of the human body to remove obstructing material from its organic domain, and to repair damages . . . should this defense action be intensified with stimulants? subdued by narcotics? confused with counter-irritants? Can nature throw off two or three burdens, more easily than one? We do not think so."
>
> — Russell Trall

One of the main goals of naturopathic hydrotherapy is to help cure disease. In the process of helping to cure disease naturopathic hydrotherapy may precipitate an intense detoxification reaction known as a healing crisis. The concept of "healing crisis" has always been central to the naturopathic philosophy of cure. It is fitting and necessary then that we study the healing crisis in some detail.

What is a healing crisis? Rausse gives the simplest definition. He considers disease to be the result of the accumulation of morbific matter, or toxins, in the body. A healing crisis is the process by which these toxins are eliminated by the body and a cure effected.

Lindlahr gives a more complete understanding. He says, "Every acute disease is the result of a cleansing and healing effort of Nature." However, when nature is prevented from carrying out its cleansing efforts by suppressive treatments, such as drugs, a chronic disease results. Such chronic disease is cured when it is brought back to the acute stage from which it originated. This reappearance of the acute disease and the consequent elimination of the toxic matter constitute the healing crisis. A disease crisis is an acute state wherein the disease factors are in the ascendency and are overwhelming the resistance of the vital force which is on the defensive. Such a crisis may result in permanent organ damage or even death. A healing crisis, on the other hand, is an acute reaction wherein the vital force is on the offensive and able to overcome the toxic manifestations of disease. It always results in an improved condition. Clearly, it is of utmost importance that the practitioner be able to distinguish between a disease crisis and a healing crisis. This is done by being thoroughly familiar with the natural course of diseases (pathology), which is beyond the scope of our discussions, and being thoroughly familiar with the signs and symptoms of healing crises which we will discuss shortly.

Is a healing crisis necessary for cure? There is some controversy as to whether or not a healing crisis is necessary and/or desirable for the cure of disease. Rausse and Lindlahr found it a common and frequently necessary occurrence. Jackson disagreed, as did Tilden who said that under rational care a healing crisis was a rare development. Kellogg's belief that a healing crisis was the result of too strong a treatment supported their view. Homeopathic physicians have much to say on the issue because of the strong identity between the naturopathic healing crisis and the homeopathic aggravation. Many people consider them the same thing. Kent and his devotees, such as Vithoulkas, consider the homeopathic aggravation an integral part of cure, while homeopaths such as Dr. Eizyaga, who have broken from the Kentian tradition, feel that the aggravation is neither necessary nor desirable, and they use low potency remedies to keep the intensity of cure below the crisis level. While we do not deny that cure can occur without crisis, clinical experience shows that the healing crisis is a natural and frequently seen part of the healing process. We believe, therefore, that naturopathic practitioners must be able to recognize and cooperate with the healing forces represented by a crisis and to guide their patients safely through this critical passage on the road back to good health.

How is a healing crisis produced? A healing crisis, being a natural part of the body's self-regulating mechanism, can occur on its own without any prompting. However, given the stresses of modern living and the history of suppressive treatments many patients bring to the doctor's office, the human organism frequently needs skillful coaching to bring its healing forces to bear on its illness.

Healing crises can be produced only by building up the vitality of the patient and by detoxifying the patient which, of course, are mutually reinforcing activities. Homeopaths use the correctly prescribed homeopathic remedies to produce crises. Hygienists use fasting. Chiropractors of days-gone-by employed full-body manipulation three times a day, five days a week for 4-6 weeks to bring on reactions, also called retracings. Priessnitz and Rausse used hydrotherapy. Kneipp added herbs; Lindlahr used all these things together and found that the synergistic effect of these modalities hastened the onset of the healing crises.

What these various methods have in common is that they strengthen the body so that it can produce and maintain elimination while at the same time promoting detoxification of the body. Once the flow of toxins into the body has been reversed by these methods, the body's own eliminative forces come into play, detoxification accelerates, and the healing crisis occurs. Constitutional hydrotherapy is a strongly restorative and detoxifying treatment. It may be used in rational combination with diet, fasting, massage, homeopathy, herbs, etc., to induce healing crises in susceptible patients.

A fine but important point should be made here concerning detoxification. There are two basic kinds of detoxification in the body: that which takes place at the organ level and that which takes place at the cellular level. While either type of detoxification would be meaningless without the other, it is important to understand that cellular detoxification is what healing and, therefore, the healing crisis, is all about. Kellogg showed experimentally that sweat from a natural fever was many times more toxic than sweat from heat or exercise. This is because sweat from exercise is detoxification at the organ level only (sweat gland), while sweat from natural fever is detoxification at both the cellular level and the organ level. Cathartics, diuretics, saunas, etc., all work primarily at the organ level and not at the cellular level. There are practitioners who, therefore, reserve the use of such substances for the healing crisis when the organs have something significant (cellular toxins) to eliminate.

Dr. Dick, for example, says to go with the body in the use of your herbs — use your diaphoretics after the body has created its own sweat rather than before. So, a healing crisis is detoxification initiated at the cellular level.

How do you know when a healing crisis is coming? There are a few general guidelines which help you predict when a healing crisis will occur in a given patient. Generally, the stronger the patient, the sooner a healing crisis may be expected; and the weaker the patient, the later a crisis would occur. This is because the healing crisis is a vital reaction, and the patient must be built up to a critical point before his body is strong enough to respond in such a manner. Correlated to this, the less serious the disease, the sooner the crisis; and the deeper the disease, the later the crisis. In seasonal terms crises come on more quickly in the late spring and summer and more slowly in the winter. In terms of different treatments, crises tend to come more quickly when multiple modalities are employed than when just a single modality is used.

Before World War II Dr. Carroll found that it took an average of 14-20 constitutional treatments to induce a healing crisis. After the war, however, he found that it took much longer. Today it takes an average of 45, and can go as high as 100, treatments to precipitate a healing crisis. This drastic change is attributed to the introduction during the last 40 years of such devitalizing factors as antibiotics, pesticides, radiation, etc. Today, a useful rule-of-thumb to follow in your practice is this: a patient following a good diet requires approximately one constitutional hydrotherapy treatment per year of age to precipitate a healing crisis. For example, a 50-year-old patient, other things being equal, would be expected to take approximately 50 constitutional treatments to reach a crisis.

A more specific means of predicting the onset of a crisis is offered by observing changes in the patient's iris. This is well-explained in the works of Dr. Bernard Jensen. Basically chronic lesions are represented in the patient's iris by dark, open spots in the normally tightly-knit fibers of the iris, in areas corresponding to the organ or body part involved. As the patient's vitality increases, these dark lesion areas are gradually filled in with white fibers. When the lesion areas are completely filled in, the organ or body part has been strengthened to the point that it can now sustain the upheaval of the healing crisis which is required for its return to full, normal function. The observant practitioner can, therefore, roughly calculate the time of crisis onset by how fast or slowly the lesion areas fill in. For example, if it took 2 months to fill the lesion area 50%, then in another 2 months the crisis would be expected. Likewise, the nature of the healing crisis may be predicted by the location of the lesion areas which are filling in. For example, if a patient's iris showed a healing lesion in the lung area to be three-quarters filled after 6 weeks of therapy, the practitioner and the patient should be prepared for a crisis in approximately 2 more weeks involving strong respiratory symptoms. Dr. Carroll was so adept at predicting the time and type of crises in his patients by this method that many of them considered him psychic.

Finally, right before a healing crisis commences, the patient feels great. When the patient comes into your office smiling and says, "Today I give you the treatment," you can expect a crisis within 48 hours. Dr. Dick's wife, Ruby, describes the patient on the brink of a healing crisis as being "as frisky as a colt in spring." This may be the physiological equivalent of the biblical truth, "Pride cometh before a fall."

How do you know when a healing crisis is in progress? Although patients often feel great right before a healing crisis, they feel terrible during the crisis. You just don't feel good when you are eliminating toxins. Although fever is not present in 100% of crises, it is the most common symptom of a healing crisis. Please refer to the lecture on fever (Chapter 10) wherein we enumerated fever's virtues as an immune system stimulant and interpreted it as a signal that the body was ready to get down to the business of detoxification and healing. With fever comes anorexia, which is quite appropriate, as the G.I. tract shuts down its nutritive function when the body temperature is elevated. Weakness is a very common general symptom as well.

Gastrointestinal tract symptoms are prominent during healing crises, as the alimentary canal is one of the primary avenues of elimination. Nausea, vomiting, flatulence, diarrhea, and a coated tongue are common. The nature of the coated tongue can offer insight into the nature of the G.I. involvement in the crisis. Dr. Bastyr says, if the tongue is completely coated to the tip, then the entire G.I. tract is involved. When the liver is involved, the back of the tongue is coated yellow, and nausea, even jaundice, should be expected. If the papilla are visible through the coating, intestinal cramping will occur. The patient in crisis may also experience strange food cravings.

Circulatory symptoms frequently seen include increased heart rate, increased blood pressure, increased heart sounds, a visible celiac pulse and cold extremities. Hemorrhoids may appear, especially if they have previously been suppressed. Congestion of the head may be expected leading to headaches, dizziness, drowsiness and mental symptoms such as irritability, depression, anxiety, sleeplessness, fear, hopelessness, strange feelings and even hallucinations. Lymphatic congestion, reflected by a swollen and painful cisterna chyli, palpable on the left of the umbilicus at the level of L_2, frequently results in edema.

Discharges, often offensive, through the skin and mucous membranes frequently reflect the radical detoxification which takes place during a crisis. Mucus and purulent secretions may come through the skin or through the nose, vagina, urethra and any body orifice. This means that boils, rashes, runny noses, heavy urinary sediment, foul perspiration, etc., may be present. These are all very good signs.

But, to return to Lindlahr's terms, how do you distinguish a healing crisis from a disease crisis — how do you know the patient is on the way to better health rather than to a poorer state of health? If the timing of the crisis conforms to the predictive measures just enumerated, you can be fairly confident that the patient has entered a beneficial crisis. But the surest and most important sign of the healing crisis is the *return of old symptoms.* This is why it is so important to have a thorough history and to quiz your patient closely about symptoms which appear during a crisis. When previously suppressed symptoms like rashes, hemorrhoids and anxiety return during a crisis, you know you are on the right track, and that, with proper management, you will have a good outcome. Here again, your knowledge of pathology and the natural course of diseases comes into play. Obviously, a bronchitis which progresses to pneumonia of one lobe and then to pneumonia of three lobes reflects a disease crisis where the patient's defenses are being overwhelmed. In a patient undergoing fasting, constitutional hydrotherapy and/or homeopathy during a crisis, the return of old disease usually lasts no more than 24 hours. However, with fewer modalities the old disease can linger longer.

The average healing crisis lasts from 4-7 days. This can be another general guideline for judging whether or not you are dealing with a healing crisis. More specifically, about halfway through the crisis several signs should start to improve, even if the patient's symptoms remain severe. First is the tongue; it will start gradually to clear, which means you are witnessing detoxification and healing. The second is the heart beat. Even if you do not get into all the subtleties discussed in the chapter on auscultation, you should be able to recognize the increased clarity and the decreased straining of the heart sounds which reflect movement toward health. The third is the spirit of the patient. Even though he or she is still miserable with headache, stomach cramps, facial rash, etc., the spirit elevates, the mood improves, the outlook becomes more optimistic, and you can be confident that physical improvements resulting from the detoxification will shortly follow.

Your best guide to judging whether your patient is in a healing crisis or disease crisis comes from your own clinical experience based on these guidelines and your preceptorships with Drs. Dick, Scott, Bastyr or other masters.

How do you manage a healing crisis? As Dr. Jensen suggests, in the proper management of a healing crisis it is not what you do but what you don't do which is most important. Therefore, if you don't know what to do, do nothing. The Hippocratic injunction, "First do no harm," has a special application to the healing crisis. In the healing crisis the body has rallied its offensive forces to action, and its defenses are down. It's like a hockey team which has pulled its goalie out of the net for a decisive offensive thrust. It is unprepared for an insult. A suppressive treatment, such as aspirin, at such a time can be disasterous, turning a healing crisis into a deeper chronic condition or even a disease crisis. The doctor's job is to guide the patient through the crisis, allowing nature, where possible, to lead the way. The body is doing the healing and cleansing. It is the practitioner's job to make sure it is not interferred with. In practical terms, this means to rest the patient in bed with no visitors and no food. Here we should quote Dr. O. G. Carroll: "When a patient comes to this cleansing period called 'Reaction,' the best advice I can offer them is to first lock all the doors and unplug the telephone. Second, keep all advisors out. Third, settle down to a total fast from all foods for four full days."

Clearly, some of the most important "management" of the healing crisis takes place before the onset of crisis in the form of educating the patient as to what to expect, so that the patient will not be scared into accepting suppressive treatments that friends, family or doctors unfamiliar with naturopathic healing principles might suggest. During the crisis "expectancy," or watchful waiting without unnecessary intervention, is indicated. The blood pressure, heart sounds, temperature, bowel sounds, tissue tone, tongue and urine should be monitored and recorded. Although a total or "dry" fast may be indicated in special instances, such as appendicitis, ample water should be taken, as a rule, by the fasting patient in crisis. Even constipated patients usually have good bowel movements during a crisis, but if the bowel does not move and impaction is suspected, an enema may be given. The patient should be rested in a quiet semi-dark room lit with natural light. There should be no running or other heavy exercise. Radio, television and reading are not recommended. Hydrotherapy should be administered in a supportive way. If strong fever is present (greater than 104 °F) and/or if elimination through the skin is great, the wet sheet pack is indicated. If fever is not high, the constitutional treatment should be done,but in one of the special sequences reserved for such instances (see page 142). Manipulation of the spine, extremities, abdomen and liver may be done as indicated. Deep breathing should not be neglected, especially in severe cases. Even in winter, the patient should be well covered and all windows opened for five minutes of deep breathing each hour. This alone can often make the difference between an easy and difficult crisis. Acute homeopathic remedies may also be applied in supportive ways if discomfort becomes great. The patient should be regularly informed as to what is being done and what is happening and why it is happening. Reassurance is important; counseling may be helpful. When the healing crisis is complete, it is important to terminate the fast properly, which we will discuss in a moment.

How do you know when the healing crisis is over? Most healing crises last a few days — Dr. Dick says from 4-7 days. Occasionally a crisis may last several weeks, and, rarely, even months. Obviously, when a crisis is over, the patient will feel and look better, but he or she may still be weak. We find that the tongue is the most accurate guide as to when the healing crisis has run its course. Just as the time of onset of the crisis may be predicted by how rapidly iris lesions fill in, so may the duration of a crisis be predicted by the rate of clearing of the coating on the tongue. If at the onset of the crisis two-thirds of the tongue's surface is covered with a yellow coating, and after three days only one-third is covered, the crisis would be expected to last three more days for a total of six days. Other important indications that the crisis is over are that discharges stop, the oral temperature goes down and stays below 99° F, and the heart sounds normalize. Mental and physical symptoms which arose during the crisis, including those which returned from old diseases, will have disappeared. Basically, if you are clinically astute enough to know when a genuine healing crisis has begun, you will have no problem telling when it has ended. Please note: in patients whose blood pressure falls below 70/50 or whose heart rate becomes less than 35 or whose oral temperature falls below 96.5° F, the fast must be broken and the crisis aborted whether it is "complete" or not.

How do you manage the patient who has completed a crisis? Once the crisis has ended, it is the clinician's job to ease the patient back toward a more normal existence. Most importantly this means ending the fast in a proper fashion and returning the patient to a nutritious diet.

The first rule in breaking a fast following a crisis is to wait at least 12 hours after the oral temperature has fallen and remained below 99° F before reintroducing nourishment. After that a number of methods may be followed.

Dr. Carroll prescribed vegetable broth for as many days after the fast as the fast lasted. In other words, a 7-day water fast would be broken by 7 days of vegetable broth. He recommended cooking ½ cup of finely cut carrots and ½ cup of finely cut celery in 2 cups of water and then giving ½ cup of the resultant broth to the patient every ½ hour as long as no nausea developed. If nausea appeared, the broth would be given at wider intervals. After the required days of broth the patient could take the cooked vegetables themselves, and, as these were tolerated, work gradually up to more substantial foods.

Dr. Dick abbreviates this considerably with good success. He uses the broth as per the above recipe, but once the first batch is taken and tolerated, he moves the patient onto the cooked vegetables, ½ cup every hour until this second batch is gone. If no ill effects occur, the patient may sequentially be given potatoes, other vegetables, grains and meats, so long as these foods do not violate his food intolerance (see Chapter 31). In chronic cases finishing a longer fast, the broth period is often extended to 24 hours.

Dr. Shelton used whole, peeled oranges for breaking fasts, 4 oz. every 2 hours from 8 a.m. to 6 p.m. the first day, 8 oz. every 2 hours during the same hours the second day and 12 oz. of orange, melon or tomato every 2 hours during the third day.

Dr. D. J. Scott in Cleveland, who has fasted over 10,000 patients, uses pure, undiluted, fresh-squeezed orange juice, 4 oz. every 3 hours the first day. On the second day 8-10 oz. of orange juice is alternated with 8 oz. of vegetable juice (carrot, celery, romaine) at 3-hour intervals. On the fourth day the normal diet is resumed. In cases of longer fasts (over 3 weeks) the period of juices-only would be extended accordingly.

Any of these methods or reasonable combinations or variations thereof would be good for breaking the healing-crisis fast. Watch the tongue and listen to the heart during the reintroduction of foods to see if you are going too quickly or in the wrong direction with the diet. And please note, the gradual reintroduction of foods to the patient who has completed a crisis would parallel the gradual reintroduction of other activities such as exercise, socializing and work — that is, gradually and as tolerated.

What are the contraindications for a healing crisis? Not every patient can go through a healing crisis. Rausse found in his practice, and this has been confirmed by others, that most patients go through healing crises except those in certain categories. The patient who is too weak cannot muster the immune forces necessary to create a fever and therefore cannot enter a healing crisis until the strength has been greatly increased through natural therapies. As many as 12-14 months may be required to do this. The patient who has received too strong a treatment also will not go into crisis, because his reactive capacities have been exceeded. The patient who is healthy and has nothing to eliminate will not go through a healing crisis. And the strong patient who, though toxic, has good daily elimination and progresses in a steady, gradual fashion, will not go into crisis.

More important are the patients who, though perhaps capable of entering a healing crisis, should never be allowed to. The healing crisis is contraindicated in fearful or neurotic patients who would be unable to cope with the additional mental, emotional and spiritual stresses of a crisis. Healing crisis is contraindicated in patients undergoing a particularly stressful period in life such as loss of a loved one or a major career change. Once these life-stresses have subsided, such a person may then be considered for therapy directed toward a healing crisis. Patients under the care or influence of others (doctors, relatives) or who "know better than you" and don't follow your instructions are *not* candidates for a healing crisis. As pointed out earlier, great harm may be done by suppressive intervention during crises. If you don't have control over the patient and cannot monitor the patient's status, do not take that patient into a crisis. Just as too many cooks spoil the broth, so do too many physicians ruin the patient. Patients whose urine specific gravity consistently remains less than 0.015 should not be taken to crisis as the kidneys cannot eliminate the toxins adequately. The other important contraindication for the healing crisis is the patient on medications, e.g., a diabetic under insulin treatment. No medication should ever be given during a healing crisis. This does not mean to take a medicated patient off his drug after inducing a crisis, but rather it means not to induce a crisis in such a patient. While withdrawal from certain addictive drugs may be accomplished in strong patients as part of a healing crisis, it would be reckless practice to withdraw a patient from a medicinal drug via the healing crisis or to precipitate a healing crisis by withdrawing the patient from his drug(s). Patients who can be successfully withdrawn from their medication(s) by other natural supportive methods such as diet and life style may then be considered for therapy leading to a healing crisis.

In conclusion, the well-managed healing crisis is not a dangerous but rather a beneficial process, akin to fever, with which the naturopathic hydrotherapist should be thoroughly familiar. The practitioner who can select appropriate patients, educate them as to what to expect, induce in them a genuine healing crisis and then guide them through it by scrupulously avoiding supressive interventions will have mastered the art of natural healing—that is, will have learned to cooperate with the healing forces of nature in its most basic healing process.

33. MANAGEMENT OF ACUTE DISEASE

"The curative effects of water depend, or may depend, largely upon combining its use with other hygienic agents."

— James C. Jackson

In this session we will articulate the general naturopathic principles for treating acute disease and then apply these principles to frequently seen acute illnesses. Since the healing crisis is an example of acute disease, many of the principles already discussed in the lecture on managing healing crises (Chapter 32) are applicable to other acute conditions. Please remember that the specific recommendations we will give for different conditions are guidelines to be used or modified as appropriate to a given case and not to be applied mechanically. We treat patients, not conditions. The guidelines offered here are intended as prompters to get your naturopathic thinking about a particular case going in the right direction. It is not the blind application of techniques but rather understanding the principles behind the techniques which allows for successful management of difficult cases. We want you to be doctors, not technicians.

The first step to take in dealing with an acute case is to diagnose the condition. This is just common-sense medicine. Do whatever physical exam or lab studies are necessary to tell you what the condition is, its expected prognosis and whether or not it is amenable to your forms of treatment.

The second step is to *fast* the patient on water. Many acute conditions are the result of a system overloaded with toxins, and fasting will facilitate the detoxification necessary for recovery. In those cases where toxicity is not a major issue, fasting will still be beneficial because it allows the body's full attention to be turned to the problem of healing rather than being siphoned off to digest and metabolize food. The fast should last until the symptoms are gone and even a few days after, if possible. Infants should not be fasted but rather may be given mother's milk or vegetable juice diluted half-and-half with pure water. No fruit juices should be taken. For how the fast should be broken, please see pages 183-184.

The third step is to administer an enema. Most acute disease involves auto-intoxication and/or fever and/or pain, and enemas can reduce all three. Enemas reduce toxicity by enhancing elimination through the bowel; cool enemas lower fever by mechanically absorbing and carrying off excess heat; enemas reduce pain by diluting kinins and other pro-inflammatory substances. There may be reflex neurological pathways involved as well. Please see Chapter 20 for instruction on the proper administration of enemas.

The fourth step is to *rest* the patient, in bed, if possible. Curtail all unnecessary exertion so that the body's full energies can be concentrated on detoxification and healing.

Fifth, employ *fresh-air breathing* five minutes each hour, especially if the patient is anxious or extremely uncomfortable. This should be done even in winter; just make sure the patient is warmly bundled before opening the windows.

Sixth, expose the patient to *ultraviolet light* which is tonic to the whole system. This is especially important in cases of infection or fracture. Sunlight is the best source, ten minutes on each side of the body, but not at the hottest time of the day during the summer. If sunlight is impractical, use your ultraviolet and your infrared lamps in the clinic. Place the UV and the IR lamps beside each other over the prone, disrobed patient so that the UV is aimed at the upper body and the IR at the lower body. Turn the lamps on for 30 seconds, then switch their positions so that the IR is over the upper body and the UV is over the lower. Again, turn lamps on for 30 seconds. Have the patient turn over to the supine position and repeat the above procedure. Determine ahead of time by strip tests the proper height of the UV lamps. See your physical therapy texts for complete instructions. Also, properly shield the patient's eyes from the UV. The UV is stimulating and the IR is soothing.

Seventh, give *appropriate massage and/or manipulation,* including trigger point therapy and spondylotherapy, to reduce pain, inflammation and swelling.

Eighth, if infection is present, employ *glandular tissue* from the immune centers such as the thymus, lymph and spleen to increase the immune response.

Ninth, apply *homeopathic* and *herbal* remedies, *acupuncture* and/or other *modalities* as appropriate and according to your expertise.

Tenth, use your *hydrotherapy* to optimize the body temperature, stimulate immunity and normalize circulation. This means you must take the temperature. If fever is present, leave it alone unless it exceeds 105° F. See Chapter 10 for proper management of fever. When the temperature is elevated, the defenses are aroused. When the temperature is depressed, the defenses are asleep. If the temperature is below normal, you must increase it.

The depressed temperature may be increased to an optimal level in several ways. One way is to give the patient a hot foot bath with mustard (see Chapter 12) for ten minutes then apply a small cold compress over the navel for ten minutes and take the temperature. A stronger measure would be to apply two hot towels over the spine of the prone patient and then to replace them via the "flip" every three minutes with two fresh hot towels, for a total of six three-minute applications. Then turn the patient over, apply a cold compress over the navel for ten minutes and check the temperature. In an exceptional case a third option may be followed — a full-body hot bath with cold compresses to the head followed by the cold compress to the abdomen. Once the temperature is optimized, apply water treatments to manipulate the circulation and boost immunity as appropriate.

These, then, are the general principles to be applied in acute cases. Let's now turn to specific acute conditions and discuss possible naturopathic hydrotherapeutic approaches to them, remembering that we are dealing in guidelines not recipes.

Otitis media or inflammation of the middle ear is a commonly seen condition, especially in children. In the office give the "42's" (see Chapter 30) and the constitutional treatment with hot and cold compresses to the affected ear corresponding to the hot and cold phases of the standard treatment. Also add an extra electrical phase to the ear. A specific home treatment to consider in otitis is the application of dry heat from a 40-watt lamp over the external ear for five minutes followed with a cold compress covered with wool for fifteen minutes. After three alternate applications of hot and cold in this manner, it is rare for the pain not to be gone. The child may fall asleep. The applications are just as effective when made behind the ear over the mastoid. Make sure not to burn the patient by holding the lamp too close. After the local hot and cold, apply heating compresses to the feet, i.e., the cold socks (see page 79). Other useful treatments include curtailing the diet, manipulation of the ear and neck, glandulars, etc. Homeopathic remedies to keep in mind would be *Belladonna* (hot, red, throbbing) *Chamomilla* (irritable, pain unendurable, one cheek red the other pale), *Kali mur* (bulging with fluid), *Ferrum phos* (before any exudate), *Mercurius* (suppurative, increased salivation), *Pulsatilla* (pale, weepy, clingy child or no clear picture).

For *sore throat* give the "42's," fast the adult patient or curtail the diet in children (see page 188), administer an enema and give the constitutional treatment, taking care to cover the throat and neck as well as the trunk with the towels. If no significant fever is present, apply short wave, preferably via a neck collar, after the treatment. If fever is a factor, apply Vita-ray (see page 155)to the external throat instead. Examine the cervical spine and make any necessary corrections. For home treatment a heating compress to the throat (see page 81) is useful, or, if pain is present, a carrot poultice may be applied to the external throat (see Chapter 23). These should be left on overnight or until dry and may be renewed as necessary. Some homeopathic remedies to consider would be *Phytolacca* (dark bluish color, ear pain with swallowing, worse night, right side, warm drinks), *Lachesis* (starts on left side, better cold drinks, worse waking), *Lycopodium* (starts on right side, better warm drinks), *Belladonna,* (sudden, hot, red, dry, from exposure to cold winds), *Hepar sulph* (chilly, sensitive to pain, better warm drinks) *Lac caninum* (changes from side-to-side, better cold drinks) and *Mercurius* as well as *Merc. sol., Merc. iod. flav.* and *Merc. iod. rub.*

Acute sinusitis requires the "42's" and fasting at the earliest possible time. Local applications or alternately hot and cold compresses (see Chapter 22) are useful so long as the hot, which could increase congestion, is not prolonged. Some of the old diathermy units have special facial pads which are very useful for sinus treatment. Nasal lavage with cold hypertonic saline (one tablespoon of salt in one quart of water), and possibly with a pinch of *Echinacea* or *Hydrastis,* should be employed. For maximum benefit pinch the nostrils shut and shake the head up and down before letting the irrigation fluid out. The first homeopathic remedy to consider in acute sinusitis is *Kali bichromium,* especially if thick, ropey mucus and a nasal voice are present. *Silicea* is strong for chronic and *Mercurius* for neglected cases. Other frequently indicated remedies are *Nux vomica, Hepar sulph, Pulsatilla, Lycopodium* and *Kali sulph.* Also, don't forget to check the upper cervical spine.

Colds and *flus* may be aborted or shortened by naturopathic care. Dr. Dick believes colds result from a chill following an unnecessary meal taken without hunger. The improperly digested food is toxic to the system, and the virus symbiotically helps the body to clean it out. At the first sign that cold or flu might be developing, the patient should take the "42 Cocktail" (see Chapter 30) and skip the next two meals. From the Drs. Thrash comes the suggestion to drink one glass of pure water every ten minutes for an hour. The body temperature should be raised via exercise, sauna, warm drinks, (e.g., yarrow tea) and/or the dry pack (like the wet sheet pack except no water is used — see Kellogg, p. 619). Of course, the constitutional hydrotherapy is well indicated, as is examination and correction of the cervical spine. Homeopathically, *Influenzinum* and *Oscillococcinum* may be given early to cut things short, and, along with *Tuberculinum,* may be given prophylactically at the beginning of the season. Once the flu is established, the homeopathic similimum should be given — *Bryonia, Eupatorium* and *Gelsemium* being common remedies to consider. The same is true for the cold, although *Mercurius, Pulsatilla* and *Nux vomica* are more commonly indicated. The frequency with which remedies are indicated in colds and flu varies from region to region.

When upper respiratory infections progress to *pneumonia,* hydrotherapy can be of great value. When fever is not a factor in pneumonia, the constitutional water treatments with "4/2" hot front and back, with diathermy over the lungs and heat to the feet is the treatment of choice (see Chapter 27). In pneumonia with significant fever, the wet sheet pack (see Chapter 25) is almost a specific. It should be applied no more than two hours at a time and no more than twice per day. It should be concluded with cold friction (see Chapter 26) which, in this and other respiratory cases, should always be applied from the feet up. If the fever is especially high, use two wet sheets, shorten the duration of the pack and do not dry the patient after the cold friction. Dr. Speisman, a colleague of Lindlahr, modified the wet sheet pack for pneumonia and was able to resolve it three to seven days faster than Dr. Lindlahr. Speisman soaked his wet sheet in magnesium sulfate (Epsom salts), used an electric blanket for his second blanket and had the patient sip hot diaphoretic teas while in the pack. The Speisman pack was applied full-body first thing in the morning for 30-45 minutes, depending on the strength of the patient. It was concluded with a dry friction rub. It was applied as a trunk pack (see Chapter 14) for 30 minutes in mid-afternoon and then right before bedtime. In between times a heating compress was applied to the chest every other hour. A brief hot application to the chest may precede each of the packs or compresses. In all cases keep the bowel open, with "42's" or enemas, if necessary. Homeopathic remedies are also useful in pneumonia, especially in conjunction with the water treatments. The stage of the disease is an important guide to the correct remedy. *Aconite, Belladonna* and *Ferrum phos* are commonly indicated in the early phase of pneumonia. Later, *Phosphorus* (especially with right lower lobe involvement) and *Bryonia* (with stitching pains eased by pressure), as well as *Ipecac, Antimonium tart,* and *Carbo veg* may be indicated. *Lycopodium* (with yellow sputum) is a later stage remedy, and *Sulphur* and *Tuberculinum* will finish up many cases, especially neglected ones. Please see

Nash's *Respiratory Leaders* and Gatchell's *Diseases of the Lungs* for a more complete discussion.

Asthma patients with an acute attack should be fasted and given the "42's." While the constitutional treatment should be given between attacks, the best treatment during a crisis is the following: a set of two folded towels (as per the constitutional treatment) as hot as possible to the chest and abdomen covered with wool for five to ten minutes; follow this with a washcloth wrung out in cold water placed unfolded over the umbilicus for 15-20 minutes covered with wool; then repeat this sequence three more times. If the attack is accompanied by anxiety, begin with several hot applications to the back and then proceed as above. In seeking a homeopathic remedy, pay attention to the position the patient assumes during an attack. Sitting erect or leaning slightly forward suggests *Arsenicum,* while leaning far forward with the head over, on or between the knees suggests *Kali carb.* Other strong remedies for acute asthma are *Lobelia, Ipecac* and *Pulsatilla.* In *Arsenicum* and *Pulsatilla* cases, be prepared for the disappearance of the asthma to result in a skin eruption. If you don't understand this, look at page 180 about suppression and retracing. Also, remember to examine the cervical and thoracic spines, including the ribs.

Those of you with a pediatric practice know that *colic* is a common problem in infants. There are simple hydrotherapies you can teach the parents which can be very helpful. Ideally the temperature of the infant should be taken during the colic attack. If the rectal temperature is above 99.6° F, a cotton washcloth wrung out in cold water and folded in quarters should be applied over the abdomen and covered with wool. If the rectal temperature is below 99.6° F, a cotton washcloth wrung out in warm water and folded in quarters should be applied over the abdomen and covered with wool, care being taken not to make the warm compress too hot. It is not always practical to take the rectal temperature of a raging infant. When the temperature is not known, start with the warm application. If it is the wrong treatment, the child will let you know. If the child gets worse or is not improved within five minutes, switch to the cool application. In conjunction with the abdominal compress, the "wet socks" (heating compresses to the feet) should be used.

This diverts blood from the abdomen to the lower extremities and reduces congestion (see Chapter 14). Homeopathic remedies to consider are *Chamomilla, Rheum, Cina, Nux vomica, Mag phos* and *Colocynthis,* the latter especially if the colic seems related to an emotional upset within the family.

For *acute food poisoning* give the "42 Cocktail," then apply the sine surge to the T_5 area for five minutes. Follow this with sine to the abdomen and the thoracolumbar junction for five minutes. Then apply the hot and cold towels five and ten minutes respectively front and back. *Arsenicum* is probably the most frequently indicated homeopathic remedy for food poisoning, although *Nux vomica, Pyrogenium, Veratrum, Kreosotum* and *Podophyllum* should be kept in mind. The hydrotherapeutic treatment for drowning and for carbon monoxide poisoning is the same as for food poisoning, except no "42 Cocktail" should be given. As a supplemental treatment in cases of suffocation, asphyxia, exhaustion, etc., a series of alternating hot and cold applications to the spine should be considered, as well as such homeopathic remedies as *Antimonium tart, Carbo veg,* and *Laurocerasus.*

Acute bowel inflammations such as *appendicitis* may not be something you would feel comfortable treating naturopathically; however, many of the old-timers took such cases routinely and with good success. Even if you would not normally touch such a case, you should be acquainted with a rational hydrotherapeutic approach to appendicitis in the event you are faced with such a case in a time or place where emergency facilities are not available. The fast is of utmost importance, and it should be a dry fast *a la* Schroth (i.e., with no fluids) until the crisis is over. An ice pack (see Chapter 19) should be applied over the appendix for 15 minutes along with a hot bath to the feet. This should be followed by a fomentation (Chapter 17), the hotter the better, over the whole abdomen for 15 minutes. Then a series of five heating compresses (Chapter 14) should be applied to the abdomen for ten minutes each. The abdominal fomentation and the heating compresses should be repeated as above until the crisis has passed. Heat to the feet should be continuous throughout these applications. Once the crisis is over, an abdominal pack and a trunk pack

(Chapter 14) should be given with an additional cold compress (such as a washcloth wrung out in cold water and folded in quarters) placed over the appendical area. The patient should be allowed sleep during this four to five hour application. A small warm-water enema should be administered at the earliest possible juncture in the treatment and repeated every six hours. Homeopathic remedies such as *Bryonia, Belladonna* and *Iris* will be helpful during the crisis, if indicated by the symptom picture.

The mustard poultice is the treatment of choice for *acute nausea* and *vomiting* which is not related to organic gastrointestinal disturbances. Good diagnosis enters here, as the mustard poultice is contraindicated in appendicitis or when cramping is present. The poultice is prepared by mixing dry mustard powder with an egg white or one tablespoon of vegetable (e.g., olive) oil till it is strong enough for the fumes to burn your eyes. Wring out a washcloth in warm water and apply the mustard preparation over one-quarter of the cloth as in the following diagram.

FIGURE 9

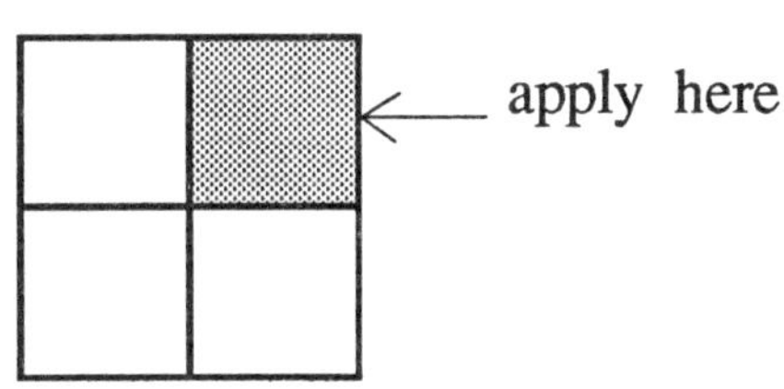

Fold the washcloth in quarters so that the mustard is on the inside. Apply the washcloth over the umbilicus so that there is only one layer of the washcloth between the mustard and the skin, then cover it with wool. Leave it in place until the skin turns pink and becomes sweaty under the compress, usually five to seven minutes, or sooner if it becomes too uncomfortable for the patient. Make sure to time the length of the application. Then apply a cold compress (a washcloth wrung out in cold water and folded in quarters would be good) over the umbilicus for exactly the same length of time as the mustard poultice. Cover with wool. Now repeat the mustard poultice (the original one may be used) until the pinkness and sweat return. This should be a shorter time, usually about four minutes. Then renew the cold compress for the length of time equal to the second mustard poultice. Repeat these applications in the same manner for a third time. This should go a long way toward stopping the nausea and/or vomiting, but the treatment may be repeated as necessary. Care must be taken not to burn the patient with the mustard. The mustard may be diluted with cornstarch in infants, one part mustard to three parts cornstarch. Dr. Dick says to leave vomiting alone so long as it is productive, but use this treatment for debilitating dry heaves. Remember, this treatment is contraindicated in appendicitis or other organic G.I. disease, or if cramping is present.

Acute meningitis is a condition most current practitioners shy away from; however, it is important that you understand the principles of hydrotherapeutic treatment in the event you are ever faced with such a case where modern facilities are not available. In meningitis, think: congestion of the brain; therefore, the hydrotherapeutic goal would be to draw blood and lymph away from the head. This would be done by applying cold to the head and neck along with warm to the rest of the body in the form of a full-body bath or wet sheet pack taken quickly to the heating stage. Treatments should be vigorous and continuous. Homeopathically, study the remedies under Kent's rubric "head, Inflammation of Brain," which includes *Aconitum, Apis, Belladonna, Cuprum, Hyoscyamus,* and *Stramonium* for the acute stage. *Opium, Helleborus* and *Zincum* are the main remedies for late stage and for sequellae. And remember *Natrum sulph* in cases which have never been well since meningitis.

Myocardial infarction and *acute angina* are other conditions the old-timers do not shrink from treating. In serious problems such as these Dr. Dick recommends always starting with the "42 Cocktail" and the sine wave machine five minutes to the T_5 area and five minutes to the abdomen and thoracolumbar region, followed by the standard hot and cold towels of the constitutional treatment without further electricity.

Listen to the heart sounds throughout the treatment and employ the "heart drops" (see page 162). Manipulation of the cervical and upper thoracic spines is also indicated, as well as consideration of *Cactus, Aconitum, Latrodectus,* and *Arsenicum.*

One class of conditions you should not be afraid of facing with hydrotherapy is tissue infection, such as *cellulitis* and *lymphangitis,* especially in the extremities of otherwise healthy patients. You should fast the patient and give the constitutional treatment with an extra electrical phase with one pad on the affected extremity distal to the infection site and the other pad on the spinal area on that side governing the corresponding dermatome. Frequent doses of Echinacea herb along with vitamin C, thymus and other immune-stimulating factors should be prescribed. Alternate hot and cold treatments (see Chapter 22) should be carried out at home. At night the heating compress in the form of the cotton glove, sleeve or sock (see Chapter 14) should be put in place at bedtime and left on until the morning. The progress of the infection should be stopped within six hours after the first treatment, otherwise it is the wrong treatment for that case. Homeopathically *Lachesis, Hypericum,* and *Arsencium* may be useful.

For *acute cystitis* the most important thing to remember is never to apply cold over the bladder. Instead, use a hot Epsom salts compress covered with wool and kept warm by a heating pad, hot water bottle or infrared lamp. The neutral sitz bath (see Chapter 16) is also indicated and may be alternated with the above. The "Bladder tea" (see page 161) should also be employed. *Cantharis* is one of the first homeopathic remedies to consider for this condition along with *Pulsatilla, Berberis, Equisetum, Sarsaparilla* and others. For *acute nephritis* remember the wet sheet pack wrung out with Epsom salts water, once per day only. Also the revulsive treatment on the back over the kidney using fomentations for the hot phases may be employed, followed by a heating compress to the abdomen. Then let the patient sleep. For glomerulonephritis *Apis, Cantharis* and *Terebenthina* are to be considered; for pyelonephritis think of *Cantharis, Berberis, Lycopodium* and *Sarsaparilla.*

For *acute gallstone or kidney stone attacks* use your hot fomentations to dilate the passage way and relax the painful tissue. Give five to ten minutes of hot followed by less than one minute of cold (ice pack is best) followed by five minutes with a cold compress. Repeat this sequence two or three times or more, if necessary. In severe cases use vinegar water for all phases of the above sequence in concentrations from one-in-ten to fifty-fifty. Renal and biliary colic come close to the worst pain patients can feel. Use your homeopathic remedies — *Lycopodium, Berberis, Pariera, Dioscorea, Nux vomica* and *Ocimum for renal colic and Lycopodium, Chelidonium, Mag mur* and *Belladonna* for biliary colic — as indicated.

For *acute tumor pain* apply the hot coffee poultice (see Chapter 23) over the affected area and cover with wool overnight. To intensify the effect make two to three alternate applications of hot and cold coffee poultices, in this case ending with the hot poultice and leaving this last one on overnight.

For *acute inflammations of the eye,* including *glaucoma, iritis, conjunctivitis, blepharitis* and *trauma,* apply a hot compress locally for one to three minutes followed by a cold potato poultice. Grate the potato, preferably a fresh red one, onto cheesecloth. Apply the cheesecloth and potato directly to the eye, cover with a washcloth wrung out in cold water and then cover this with wool. Also, use the constitutional treatment, but add an extra electrical phase of three minutes continuous sine over the temples before turning the patient over after the normal phase 3. Use your homeopathic remedies as well, *Nat mur* being the most common in iritis, *Nux vomica* the most common in chronic glaucoma, and, for acute glaucoma, study *Aconite, Gelsemium, Physostygma, Allium cepa* and *Euphrasia* first. For injuries from blows to the eye think first of *Arnica* and *Symphytum* and then *Asarum,* if they fail. For black eyes consider *Ledum* in the later stages after *Arnica.*

For *acute hypertension* give an enema and then a hot full-body bath with cold compresses to the head and neck. The blood-pressure lowering effects of this treatment can last up to six hours. Realize that this is not curative but rather a temporary measure for dealing with a crisis. Spondylotherapy to T_9 is also indicated. In acute states *Belladonna,*

Bryonia and *Gelsemium* are often called for. In resistant cases of essential hypertension which need immediate attention *Gelsemium* 1X, if you can obtain it, is probably the best remedy from our materia medica. Give it three times per day seven days per week until the blood pressure makes a significant move downward, then reduce it to just four days per week and wean completely off as soon as possible. In one study twenty-two out of twenty-two cases of high blood pressure were returned to normal within four to six weeks following such a program and were off all therapies after six months. Of course, for the long term, changes in life style are mandatory.

For *acute dental pain,* e.g., after dental surgery, fast the patient, then give the constitutional treatment with the following modifications. During the five minute hot phase on the chest and abdomen apply a hot compress on the cheek over the site of the pain, cover with wool and then apply infrared over this. During the ten minute cold phase to the chest and abdomen apply a cold compress to the cheek and leave it on an additional ten minutes during the electrical phases to the abdomen and thoracolumbar junction. After turning the patient over, apply the hot and cold to the cheek as above in the corresponding phases of the treatment of the back. After concluding the treatment give five minutes of Vita-ray locally. Consider *Arnica, Chamomilla, Hypericum,* etc. for homeopathic relief.

For *acute abscesses* there are three ways to go — dispersal, drainage or leaving it alone when unsure of the best treatment. To disperse an abscess apply hot compresses to the abscess while giving a hot and then a cold abdominal compress, five and ten minutes respectively. Then administer alternate hot and cold compresses over the abscess, making sure the heat is strong enough to produce an erythema. To bring an abscess to a head so that it may be successfully drained, apply hot Epsom salts fomentations for 15 minutes at a time and repeat as necessary until the lesion is ripe. Then open surgically and drain. Many abscesses respond to *Tarantula cub.,* especially if pain and a mottled blue color are present. Other remedies to consider are *Arsenicum* (with prominent mental symptoms) *Pyrogenium* (with fever) and *Anthracinum.* Some authors recommend using the higher potencies to disperse, and the lower potencies to bring to a head for drainage, however, the correct remedy in whatever potency would promote the most effective reaction.

For *acute joint inflammations,* such as *arthritis* and *bursitis,* fast the patient and administer an enema. If the joint feels hot, apply local heat only briefly as part of a series of alternating hot and cold applications. If fever is present, give the Epsom salts wet sheet pack. As the inflammation is reduced and the subacute phase is entered, i.e., when the joint no longer feels hot, have the patient rub the involved area every night with Epsom salts until it becomes slippery (see Chapter 21) while in a hot bath. This opens the pores. Then dry off and rub castor oil or peanut oil or Egyptian oil (Edgar Cayce's) liberally into the area, then cover with a heating compress and go to bed for the night (see Chapter 14). For acute bursitis consider *Apis, Bryonia* and *Belladonna,* and for sub-acute and chronic, consider *Natrum mur, Ruta, Silicea,* and *Sticta.*

For *acute hemorrhoids* employ positive galvanism. Cover a *wooden* (never metallic) chair with a dry folded towel then cover the positive galvanic electrode with a moist compress (such as a 4'' x 4'') and have the patient sit on the compress so that it is in contact with the hemorrhoidal tissue. Put the negative electrode on the leg or back. Give five minutes of stimulation at 5-15 milli-amps or about one milli-amp per square inch or less, then follow with the constitutional treatment. To increase the effectiveness, moisten the electrode compress with witch hazel. Homeopathic suppositories from Boericke and Tafel or other good pharmacies can be helpful. For bleeding piles use *Hypericum* tincture 10 drops three to four times per day locally. Stool softeners such as powdered psyllium seed will prevent further unnecessary irritation. *Hamamelis, Aesculus, Muriatic Acid, Ratanhia* and *Collinsonia* are good acute homeopathic remedies to consider. *Nux vomica, Sulphur, Sepia* and other constitutional remedies with strong hepatic effects should be considered in your follow-up. In cases of *acute prostatitis* the same positive galvanic treatment may be given.

For *acute hemorrhage,* e.g., nose, uterus, lung, but not the lower extremities, give a hot foot bath (Chapter 12) for ten minutes. Two minutes after the hot foot bath has started, apply a cold compress over the area of bleeding and cover with a single thickness of wool for 20 minutes. If available, an ice pack applied for 10 minutes would be even better than the compress. Repeat the above process, up to three times, if needed. Also employ the measures described in Chapter 8 on the control of circulation as appropriate, e.g., apply long cold to the spinal and other reflex zones related to the bleeding area. Bayberry bark tea is a good herbal remedy to employ at the same time. *Ipecac, Ferrum phos,* and *Millifollium* are homeopathic remedies to consider.

For *acute pelvic inflammatory disease (PID)* and also for *ovarian cysts* and *uterine fibroids* the black salve vaginal pack has long been used in conjunction with the constitutional treatment. To prepare a vag pack, open up a "4x4" gauze pad to two thicknesses, place a tablespoon of black salve (see page 164) inside, then close it and tie it with dental floss. Clip off any extra gauze below the tie, and leave enough floss so that a few inches will protrude from the vaginal opening once the pack is in place to facilitate removal. Insert the pack gently through a properly placed vaginal speculum and position it deep into the vagina so that it is in contact with the cervix. If necessary, cotton or lamb's wool may be packed in as well to hold the black salve in place. After the vag pack is in place, give the standard constitutional treatment, and finish with five minutes of diathermy to the pelvic area. On the following day repeat the constitutional treatment and diathermy, leaving the pack in place. Instruct the patient to remove and dispose of the vag pack the following morning upon rising. That afternoon or evening insert a new pack and give the regular hydrotherapy and diathermy. The next day give the hydrotherapy and diathermy, leaving the pack alone. Have the patient remove the pack the next morning. Then put in a new pack later in the day followed by the hydrotherapy and diathermy. Continue this sequence, i.e., removal and renewal of the vag pack every two days, except during menstruation, for three to six months, if necessary. Of course, attend to the diet, life style and other pertinent factors.

Hydrotherapy has a great role to play in the enhancement of athletic performance and the prevention and treatment of *athletic injuries.* Kellogg did many experiments which showed that brief hot showers followed by brief cold showers greatly enhanced work performance if given before the activity and, if given after, significantly speeded recovery in persons exhausted by prolonged exercise. When used in conjunction with massage, the results of these showers can be even more dramatic. For extreme exhaustion as, e.g., in a marathon runner, one dose of *Arnica* 10M may also be given. For *sprains* and *strains* in the acute phase use the ice pack (see Chapter 19) along with rest, compression, elevation and homeopathic *Arnica* 30C given as frequently as every two hours. In the subacute phase use alternate baths (see Chapter 22), centripedal massage and raw onion poultices (see Chapter 23). Paint the injured area with *Arnica* tincture before taping. Consider *Rhus tox, Ruta* or *Ledum* if large ecchymoses or swelling persists. Consider *Calcarea carb* for weak joints, *Strontium carb* for the tendency to re-sprain the same joint and *Ammonium mur* for contractures, e.g., Dupuytren's. For *muscle spasms* employ formentations (see Chapter 17).

In closing it is important to note that some acute crises can be avoided by preventative intervention. The area of obstetrics offers good examples, and we will mention some naturopathic treatments to help insure healthy pregnancies and easy deliveries. First of all, if possible, make sure the prospective parents are in top health before they even try to conceive a child. This is especially important to remember in cases of infertility, which often respond to naturopathic treatment. After conception Dr. Carroll used five constitutional treatments, all in the same week, sometime during the third month of pregnancy, to help lift the uterus out of the pelvis, thus preventing nausea due to malposition and varicose veins due to congestion. He then repeated these five treatments during a week in the seventh month of pregnancy, all sine pads being kept above the level of the uterus, to prepare for labor. He also used the "Pregnancy Tea" (see page 161). Reportedly, his patients had uneventful pregnancies and deliveries. Dr. Dick uses ten treatments within two weeks during the third month and ten treatments within two weeks during the seventh month. Dr. Bastyr recommends using the blue cobalt light, 500 to 1000 watts, for ten minutes 18 inches above the bare, pregnant abdomen followed by a cold abdominal compress for

15 minutes. The same treatment is then given to the back. He uses this once a week during the last six months of pregnancy to tonify and strengthen the tissues. He also recommends alternating hot (4-6 min.) and cold (½-1 min.) sitz baths (see Chapter 16) at bedtime at least once, and up to three times, per week during the last months of pregnancy. His record as an obstetrician speaks for itself. Also don't forget to make sure the sacroiliac joints are mobile throughout the pregnancy and at the onset of labor, using manipulation whenever necessary. The importance of this cannot be overemphasized. If you are a naturopath doing home births and are not manipulating your patients' pelves, you are offering incomplete care and risking many unnecessary trips to the emergency room (and operating room) for complications arising out of failure to progress. *Cimicifuga* 30C has been successfully used during the seventh and ninth months to prepare the uterus for efficient labor, and should be considered unless other remedies are indicated. *Caulophyllum* 30 or 200 can be given at the onset of labor to insure its progress to a productive conclusion. Don't forget *Pulsatilla* for a malpositioned fetus.

34. MANAGEMENT OF CHRONIC DISEASE

> "True Materia Medica: First, air; second, food; third, water; fourth, sunlight; fifth, dress; sixth exercise; seventh, sleep; eighth, rest; ninth, social influence; tenth, mental forces."
>
> — James C. Jackson

From Lindlahr's point of view chronic disease is the result of suppression of acute disease, i.e., the result of thwarting, through drugs and other means, the body's attempt to detoxify itself. In these classical naturopathic terms, the goal of chronic disease management is to bring the chronic condition back to the acute stage, i.e., to strengthen the vital force so that it can mount a healing crisis and finally deal properly with the problem which was originally suppressed.

In this regard the principles of management of chronic disease are similar to those for the management of acute disease, although some of the emphases are different due to the less pressing nature of chronic conditions as opposed to acute ones. Many successful strategies are possible. We will present a strategy commonly employed by naturopathic physicians who make great use of hydrotherapy.

The first principle of naturopathic treatment of chronic conditions is to *do no harm. Primum non nocere.* This means to discard or reject any treatment or diagnostic technique which can cause harm unless absolutely necessary. Granted, any treatment, when done improperly, can do harm. But we are talking about treatments which can do harm even when done correctly.

Second, *seek and remove external causes,* e.g., toxic working conditions, drug use, geopathic stresses, lack of exercise, etc. Dr. Lindlahr did a lot of work with the miners from the Illinois coal fields. He would tell them,"You don't need a doctor, you need a new job." It is not always so simple as this, yet sometimes it is, and we must be vigilant in this regard so that we don't miss easy cures.

Third, *attend to the nutrition.* The first half of this is to remove the injurious foods — those which are unhealthy in general (junk foods, like candy and potato chips, and hard-to-digest foods, such as peanut butter, shellfish, pork and processed cheese) and those which are found to be specifically harmful to an individual patient who is intolerant to them (see Chapter 31). The second half is to feed the nutritious foods — whole foods, in season, grown locally on good soils — and correct any nutritional imbalances with dietary supplements, if necessary.

Fourth, *detoxify the patient.* Dr. Dick's immortal words cannot be repeated too often. "Detoxification is the name of the game." Detoxification is not a metaphor: it is a biochemical fact and necessity. The patient will not get better until the toxic stumbling blocks are removed so that the *Vis Medicatrix Naturae* can do its job. Detoxify the patient through fasting, hydrotherapy, homeopathy, breathing, exercise, herbs, clay, charcoal, massage, manipulation and/or nutrition, as appropriate. Of course, we feel the constitutional hydrotherapy is one of the most effective methods for promoting detoxification.

Fifth, *prescribe the indicated homeopathic remedies,* one at a time as classically taught by Hahnemann in the *Organon of Medicine.* Homeopathic treatment is essential for permanent cure because it can remove the most important cause of disease, the abnormal susceptibility.

Sixth, *correct any musculoskeletal defects,* i.e., subluxations, adhesions, fixations, etc., through massage, manipulation, physical therapy, neural therapy, acupuncture, etc.

Seventh, *educate the patient* to maintain his or her improved health and prevent recurrence of old disease or development of new disease by rational use of the previous six principles.

Each case is different, but these are the general principles which should be applied in specific ways as appropriate to each patient. These principles represent the context within which we operate as naturopathic hydrotherapists.

The two most important techniques compatible with these principles are the food intolerance diet (see Chapter 31) and the constitutional hydrotherapy (see Chapter 27). They are the therapeutic cornerstones in the management of chronic disease along with a third modality, *patience.* The natural treatments are effective, but they take time. Dr. Dick had an eczema patient that required 100 treatments to cure. He had to treat one psoriasis patient for a year-and-a-half before cure was achieved. Consequently, he has adopted the practice of giving the first patient consultation free of charge to explain the principles of naturopathic medicine and make sure the patient understands that natural cures require the responsible participation of the persevering patient.

By this time the proper application of the techniques and principles we have been teaching for chronic conditions should be fairly self-evident, and it would be unnecessarily redundant to run through chronic disorders disease-by-disease. Instead, we will discuss some special considerations in the management of a couple of commonly encountered chronic conditions.

Diabetes is a good disease with which to begin. Here the diet and the constitutional treatments are of utmost importance, but the real management problem comes in monitoring the blood glucose and insulin needs which may change drastically in response to these treatments. Most natural therapies in general and the constitutional hydrotherapy in particular potentiate any allopathic medications a patient may be taking. This is because the constitutional treatments improve the body's overall functioning and make less drug necessary to influence a certain aspect of the metabolism. This is a very important point for you to grasp. When the natural therapies are successful in the medicated patient, it is very easy to get into an overdose situation if the medications are not monitored and, when appropriate, lowered. For diabetics on insulin you must check the blood sugar levels before the constitutional treatment, immediately after the treatment and then again two hours after the treatment. In most cases you will see a considerable reduction in blood sugar levels between the before-and after-treatment readings. If no such reduction occurs, the medication should not be adjusted. However, if the expected reduction in blood glucose occurs, then the third reading becomes critical. If it has not risen significantly over the second reading and is not over 170 mg/dl, you may consider cutting the insulin dosage by one-quarter to one-half. Monitoring the blood glucose like this daily until a reliable stability is achieved will prevent a possibly serious hypoglycemic crisis as a side effect to your successful treatments. Some advanced cases may require 24-hour monitoring at first. Dr. Dick says it is more difficult to cure diabetes if the patient has been habituated to insulin for a long time. However, it is possible to lower the insulin requirements in almost all medicated diabetics, and this is important as a preventive measure because of the side effects of insulin. Of course, for legal reasons, adjustments in the prescription medications of any of your patients will be made by a physician licensed to prescribe. Also, remember the homeopathic remedies — *Phosphorus, Phosphoric Acid,* etc. — as well as exercise, GTF chromium, pyridoxine alpha-ketoglutarate, and the contraindications — no whole-body heat or heat to the extremities in diabetics and no complete fasting.

Arthritis is another good example of a chronic condition we can discuss. Again the food intolerance and constitutional treatments are paramount, but there are some other things to consider. Joint problems offer many occasions for adding extra phases to the constitutional treatment, e.g., three minutes of continuous sine to the arthritic knee and the spinal area governing the dermatome to the knee after the normal 3rd phase. In chronic cases such extra phases of localized treatments (see pages 142-143) should not be started until the patient has received at least five standard constitutional treatments. Many arthritis patients suffer from what we have referred to as the "rheumatic diathesis." A great percentage of these people tend to be chilly and poorly reactive to cold. Thus they require extra sets of hot towels, e.g., the "½" (see page 141), and their cold towels should be wrung out drier, and they may need extra covers to keep them warm during the cold phases. Make sure you have plenty of blankets on hand. Local heating compresses to affected joints can play important roles as supplemental home treatments (see Chapter 14). Remember the local Epsom salts massage and oil pack described for acute joints (see page 199).

Rheumatoid arthritis patients will often be highly medicated on aspirin and/or Prednisone. Those who have been on prednisone for a long time are tough cases. This drug is toxic to all systems of the body, especially the immune system. Your goal is to slowly wean them off the Prednisone. You do this by selecting the indicated homeopathic remedy based on the arthritic symptoms, especially the ones present prior to their suppression by the Prednisone. *Pulsatilla, Rhus tox, Kalmia, Lycopodium, Guaiacum* and *Rhododendron* are prominent remedies to consider. Give the remedy in the 6C potency frequently — up to five times a day or more, if necessary. Remember, in Prednisone cases *there will always be exacerbations.* You and your patient should be prepared for this. Work up slowly through the 12th, 30th and 200th potencies, etc., then, as the symptoms further decrease, the Prednisone and other drugs should be taken only when needed. Fasting is often necessary in addition to the other nutritional measures. Constitutional treatment should be applied daily. The inevitable exacerbations will eventually subside and not come back, but persistence is very important in overcoming the pathological complex made up of the natural disease and the disease created by the drug(s). Again, dosage changes in prescription drugs will be made, in such cases, by a doctor licensed to prescribe.

We could go on with many more examples. Basically,the successful management of chronic cases involves the common sense applications of the principles and techniques we have been articulating all along.

In closing we might mention that correct use of hydrotherapy has an important role to play in the prevention of disease, both chronic and acute. On one hand prolonged hot applications in the form of warm baths, showers, hot tubs, etc., should be avoided because of their depressing effect on circulation, tissue tone and the immune and nervous systems which can lead to varicosities, premature aging, frequent colds, fatigue, and mental sluggishness. On the other hand cold applications in the form of cool showers, cold friction rubs, barefoot walking in the morning dew or fresh snow, and wet socks at night are bracing treatments which can enhance immunity against colds and flu, increase energy and stress tolerance and improve mental and physical performance.

35. CONSTITUTIONAL HYDROTHERAPY IN OFFICE PRACTICE

OFFICE LAY-OUT

It is beyond the scope of this course to give detailed schematics for installation of hydrotherapy equipment. If you are interested in establishing an elaborate hydrotherapy department with various douches and baths, please see Baruch's chapter on "Hydriatic Installment" in his *An Epitome of Hydrotherapy,* and find a good plumber.

We briefly discussed elsewhere about basic equipment and materials needed for hydrotherapy (see page Chapter 11) Here we would like to go over one possible floor plan (based on Dr. Harold Dick's clinic) which works well in a practice centered around constitutional hydrotherapy. Please note the diagram (Figure 10) on the next page.

FIGURE 10
OFFICE LAY-OUT FOR CONSTITUTIONAL HYDROTHERAPY

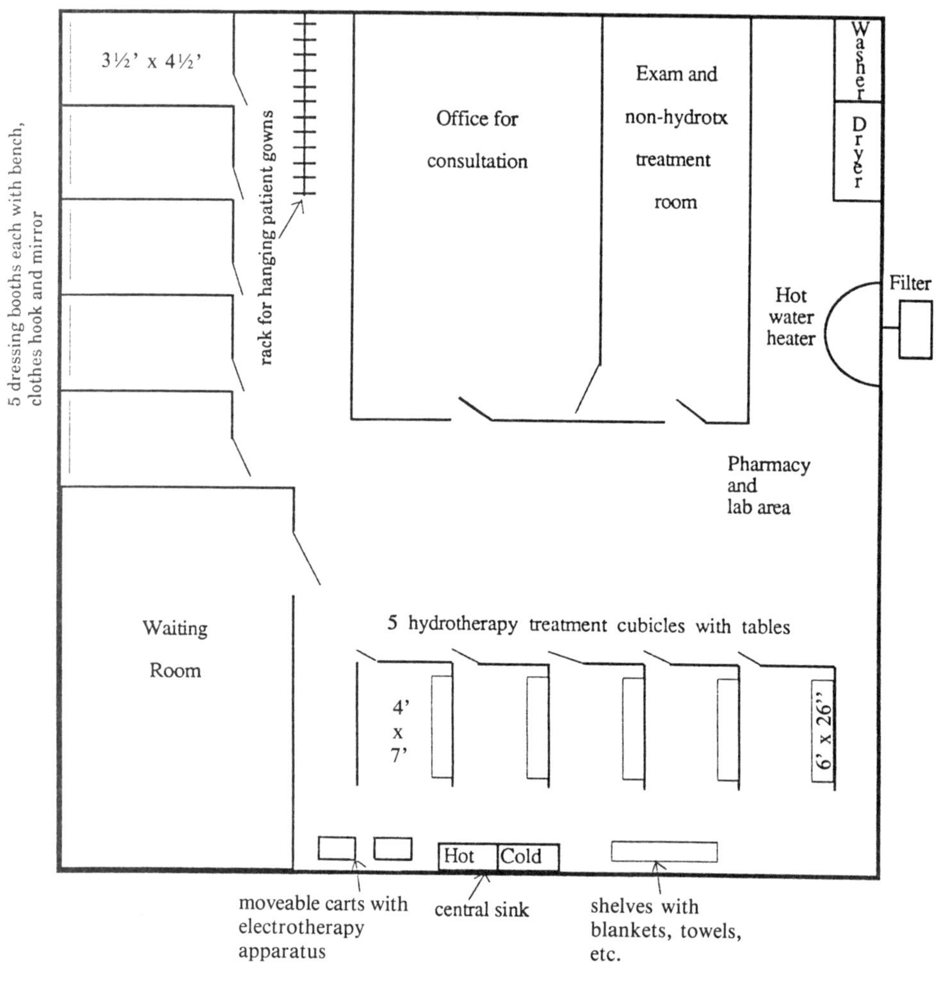

The above plan shows the patient waiting room, the doctor's office for consultation and an adjoining room for doing physical exams and non-hydrotherapy treatments. The left-hand side of the drawing shows the minimum of five dressing rooms, although you may have 8-10 or more, each equipped with a bench, clothes hooks and mirrors. Nearby is a rack upon which hang the patients' gowns, each with a patient's name on the hanger tag. These should be laundered at least once per week. The patient comes in, picks up his or her gown, enters a dressing room, disrobes, puts on the gown, then goes to a designated treatment cubicle. There are five treatment cubicles with tables across from the doctor's office separated by light-opaque partitions. Ideally these would have two-way swinging doors on the side toward the consultation office. The clinic is set up to give five constitutional treatments per hour which is just right for an adept technician. The hot and cold water sink and towels and blankets are centrally located so that the technician can minimize the time and distance he or she must travel. The sine-wave unit(s) may be on moveable cart(s) or centrally located with controls in each booth. With such a setup the doctor would spend 5-10 minutes each hour examining the patients scheduled for that hour and prescribing their treatment for the day. The rest of the time he or she can spend consulting with and examining new patients.

A good automatic washer and dryer should be located on the premises. A large capacity hot water heater is a must. Room for pharmacy and lab may be claimed as needed from the remaining floor space.

This is by no means the only workable plan for such a practice, but it gives you a point of departure for designing something suited to your needs.

PRESCRIPTION WRITING AND RECORD KEEPING

When you have dozens of patients involved in extensive constitutional hydrotherapy regimes, concise, accurate record keeping is a must. This can be combined with concise, accurate prescription writing for the hydrotherapy treatments.

The following is a form similar to the ones we used at the hydrotherapy clinic at National College of Naturopathic Medicine for charting the treatments.

CONSTITUTIONAL APPROACH

Patient Name ______________________________ Phone ______________________________

Referring Doctor ____

Symptoms and/or Diagnosis

Food Intolerance ______________________ Bad Combination ______________________

		1	2	3	4	5	6	7	8	9	10	11	12	13	14	15
Date																
Temperature Before																
Temperature After																
Sp. Gravity Before																
Sp. Gravity After																
Heart Sounds																
Bowel Sounds																
Palpation																
Herbs																
Remedies																
Other Tx																
Abdomen	Hot															
	Cold															
Chest	Hot															
	Cold															
Back	Hot															
	Cold															
Neck	Hot															
	Cold															
Feet	Hot															
	Cold															
Sitz	Hot															
	Cold															
Colonic																
Other																
Sine Wave	Dorsal															
	Lumbar															
	Solar Plexus															
	Liver															
	Spleen															
	Sm. Intestine															
	Colon															
	Pelvis															
	Other															
Diathermy	Chest															
	Abdomen															
	Other															
High Frequency																
Galvanic																
Ultraviolet																
Infrared																
Other																
Comments																
Initials																

OFFICE PRACTICE

	Standard Treatment			Chilly Patient			Healing Crisis			Healing Crisis			Foot Injury		
	1	2	3	4	5	6	7	8	9	10	11	12	13	14	15
Date															
Temperature Before															
Temperature After															
Sp. Gravity Before															
Sp. Gravity After															
Heart Sounds															
Bowel Sounds															
Palpation															
Herbs															
Remedies															
Other Tx															
Abdomen Hot	1			1/$\frac{4}{2}$			5			4			1		
Cold	2			2			6			5			2		
Chest Hot	1			1/$\frac{4}{2}$			5			4			1		
Cold	2			2			6			5			2		
Back Hot	4			4/$\frac{4}{2}$			1			1			5		
Cold	5			5			2			2			6		
Neck Hot															
Cold															
Feet Hot				2											
Cold															
Sitz Hot															
Cold															
Colonic															
Other															
Sine Wave Dorsal	2			2			3			5			2		
Lumbar	3			3			4			3			3		
Solar Plexus	3			3			4			3			3		
Liver															
Spleen															
Sm. Intestine															
Colon															
Pelvis															
Other L. foot													4		
Diathermy Chest															
Abdomen															
Other															
High Frequency															
Galvanic															
Ultraviolet															
Infrared															
Other															
Comments															
Initials															

Each numbered vertical column on the chart represents a patient's visit to the clinic. The examining physician indicates his or her prescription for that day's hydrotherapy by placing numbers corresponding to the phases of the constitutional treatments in the appropriate boxes of that day's columns showing what modality is to be applied, and where, during each phase. For example, if the first phase of the treatment consists of hot to the chest and abdomen, then a "1" is placed in the box beside "Abdomen Hot" and in the box beside "Chest Hot." If the second phase consists of cold to the chest and abdomen along with sine wave to the T_5 area, then a "2" is placed in the box beside "Abdomen Cold," and in the box beside "Chest Cold" and also in the box beside "Sine Wave Dorsal." If the third phase of the treatment consists of sine wave to the lumbar area and the small intestine,then a "3" is placed in the box beside "Sine Wave Lumbar" and in the box beside "Sine Wave Sm. Intestine." And so forth.

As examples, column #1 has been filled in with the prescription for the standard constitutional hydrotherapy treatment. Column #3 has been filled in with the prescription for a chilly patient. Those boxes marked "1/4/2" and "4/4/2" in this prescription indicate that the double application of hot towels, first for 4 minutes then for 2 minutes (see page 141) is to be employed during the first and fourth phases. Columns #7 and 10 show prescriptions suitable for patients in healing crises. Column #13 shows a prescription for a patient with an ankle problem.

The rest of the form is self-explanatory. Use of this or a similar form is vital to any clinic extensively involved in providing constitutional hydrotherapy. You may modify this for your own purposes or create your own quick charting system.

INTRODUCING PATIENTS TO HYDROTHERAPY

It is often desirable to have a printed handout describing the basics of constitutional hydrotherapy to new patients. This falls under the category of "Inform patient as to nature and rationale of treatment" which we list in the demonstrations of the techniques. The following is a copy of the handout we used at the NCNM hydrotherapy clinic.

Again, this may serve as a starting point for you to shape as you wish according to your practice needs.

HYDROTHERAPY CLINIC

Dear Patient,

Welcome to the Hydrotherapy Clinic. The Portland Naturopathic Clinic is now offering our patients the opportunity to receive constitutional hydrotherapy treatment on a regular basis. These constitutional treatments stimulate healing by enhancing the oxygenation and circulation of blood and lymph, by promoting better digestion of food and nutrition to the cells, by increasing the oxidation and elimination of toxins, by strengthening the general defense of the body and by assisting in the restoration of nervous equilibrium. Patients of all ages can benefit from these treatments.

To receive these treatments you must first be referred by your physician. A treatment session involves an initial examination by the doctor on duty of your heart, abdomen, temperature and urine. Student doctors will then fulfill the doctor's prescription by applying a series of hot and cold towels to your chest, abdomen and back, covering you with wool blankets and applying a form of mild electrical muscle stimulation. This requires that you momentarily expose your chest and abdomen at different times. Please let the doctor know if you are uncomfortable with any aspect of the procedure. Each treatment lasts approximately one hour. A doctor will be present at all times. We have five supervising physicians who each practice one evening per week. The student doctors rotate on a daily basis. After each treatment, please confirm the time of your next appointment. You are more than welcome to offer your comments and suggestions to improve this clinic in our limited facility.

During a course of hydrotherapy treatments, a person may experience fever, aches, pains, fatigue, and other discomforts, or a return of old symptoms, which are commonly encountered as a result of eliminating and healing processes. This beneficial sign of healing is called a reaction, or a healing crisis.

If any of these discomforts are occurring, please contact your physician or one of the supervising hydropathic physicians before using any measure (including aspirin), which might interfere with the natural elimination process and which could be more detrimental than helpful. Remember — if you experience a reaction, you should not treat yourself without the advice of your naturopathic physician, who is trained to guide you through a reaction and toward the subsequent improvement of your health. Remember, at all times that only nature heals and that these treatments only assist your natural healing forces.

Thank you for the privilege of serving you.

36. CONCLUSION

We have tried to give you a broad sample of the therapeutic possibilities of water and the principles upon which they are based. While we have more than "scratched the surface," we have by no means exhausted the possibilities of hydrotherapy in the naturopathic practice. For those among you who may want more, we refer you to Kellogg's *Rational Hydrotherapy* which goes into great detail concerning a variety of water treatments we were unable to discuss or could only mention briefly. We urge those of you who want to make hydrotherapy a substantial part of your practice to seek out and buy Kellogg's book. In it you will find the answer, in one form or another, to almost any hydrotherapy question which arises.

Having successfully completed this course, you should be able to face with confidence many conditions you will encounter daily in practice. Hydrotherapy offers you a wonderful opportunity to help almost every patient you see. Please do not waste this opportunity, because you do so at the expense of your patients' well-being and of your own professional growth as a clinician.

Naturopathic medicine was founded on the practice of hydrotherapy. This was not an accident of history but rather a logical — even inevitable — development, given the importance of water among the natural forces available for healing. As mentioned at the outset of this course, a certain prejudice exists against hydrotherapy, even within the naturopathic profession, because it is old, cumbersome and time-consuming, but with assistance from you, as its skilled practitioners, hydrotherapy will retain its rightful place at the heart of naturopathic medicine in helping patients get well in accordance with the precepts of nature.

With our thanks for your attention and participation we conclude this course.

BIBLIOGRAPHY

Austin, Phylis and Agatha M. and Calvin L. Thrash, *Natural Remedies: A Manual,* Seale, Alabama: Yuchi Pines Institute, 1983.

Baruch, Simon, *An Epitome of Hydrotherapy,* Philadelphia: W. B. Saunders Co., 1920.

______, "Hydrotherapy and Mineral Springs," pp. 453-533, in *A System of Practical Therapeutics,* Hobart Amory Hare, ed., Philadelphia: Lea Brothers and Co., 1891.

______, *The Principles and Practice of Hydrotherapy,* New York: William Wood and Company, 1898.

______, *The Uses of Water in Modern Medicine,* Detroit: Geo. S. Davis, 1892.

Bastyr, John, *Notes on Natural Therapeutics,* Portland: National College of Naturopathic Medicine, 1977.

Bedortha, N., *Practical Medication, or The Invalid's Guide: with Directions for the Treatment of Disease,* Albany: Munsell and Rowland, 1860.

Beni-Barde, *Traite Theorique et Pratique D'Hydrotherapie,* Paris: Libraire de l'academie de Medecine, 1874.

Brown, C., et al., "Renal Calcium and Magnesium Handling in Water Immersion in Nephrotic Patients," *Nephron,* 33: 17-20, 1983.

Bruggemann, W., *Kneipp Vademecum Pro Medico,* Wurzburg: Sebastian Kneipp Publications, 1982.

Buchman, D., *The Complete Book of Water Therapy,* New York: E. P. Dutton, 1979.

Campion, Margaret Reid, *Hydrotherapy in Pediatrics,* Rockville, Md: Aspen Systems, 1985.

Cayleff, Susan E., *Wash and Be Healed,* Philadelphia: Temple University Press, 1987.

Currie, James, *Medical Reports, on the Effects of Water, Cold and Warm, as a Remedy in Fever and Other Diseases,* Philadelphia: James Humphreys, and Benjamin and Thomas Kite, 1808.

Dick, Harold, *Hydrotherapy Seminar,* (Videotapes) Portland: National College of Naturopathic Medicine, 1983.

Erdman, Frederick, *Control of the Circulation,* Philadelphia: The Frederick Erdman Association, 1956.

Falk, Leslie A., "Black Abolitionist Doctors and Healers, 1810-1885," *Bulletin of the History of Medicine,* 54: 258-272, 1980.

Fey, Christian and Heinrich Lampert, *Hydrotherapie,* Heidelberg: Verlag fur Medizin Fischer, 1978.

Finnerty, G. B. and J. Corbitt, *Hydrotherapy,* New York: Ungar Publishing Co., 1960.

Franchimont, P., J. Juchmes and J. Lecomte, "Hydrotherapy — Mechanisms and Indications," *Pharmacology and Therapeutics,* 20 (1): 79-93, 1983.

Francke, H., *Outlines of a New Theory of Disease Applied to Hydropathy, Showing that Water is the Only True Remedy,* New York: Wiley and Halsted, 1856.

Gerberich, Susan G. and J. D. Priest, "Treatment for Lateral Epicondylitis: Variables to Recovery," *British Journal of Sports Medicine,* 19 (4): 224-227, December, 1985.

Gollard, Ann, "Basic Hydrotherapy," *Physiotherapy,* 67 (9): 258-62, September, 1981.

Greentree, L. B., "Auricular Fibrillation: An Unusual Experience," *New England Journal of Medicine,* 315 (26): 1680-1681, December 25, 1986.

Griffin, James E. and Terence C. Karselis, *Physical Agents for Physical Therapists,* Springfield, Illinois: Charles C. Thomas, 1978.

Harrison, R. A., "Tolerance of Pool Therapy by Ankylosing Spondylitis Patients with Low Vital Capacities," *Physiotherapy,* 67 (10): 296, October, 1981.

Hinsdale, Guy, *Hydrotherapy,* Philadelphia: W. B. Saunders, 1910.

Houghton, Roland S., *Bulwer and Forbes on the Water-Treatment,* New York: Fowlers and Wells, 1851.

Jackson, James, C., *Consumption: How to Prevent It and How to Cure It,* Boston, B., Leverett Emerson, 1862.

______, "Diptheria, Its Causes, Treatment and Cure," Yates County *Chronicle,* Thursday, January 25, 1863.

______, *How to Treat the Sick Without Medicine,* Dansville, New York: Austin, Jackson and Co., Publishers, 1874.

Jagger, M. and D. Zmood, "Hydrotherapy by Physiotherapists in a Community Health Centre," *Australian Family Physician,* 13 (12): 878-881, December, 1984.

Keller, Jeanne, *Healing With Water,* New York: Parker Publishing Co., Inc., 1968.

Kellogg, J. H., *Rational Hydrotherapy,* Philadelphia: F. A. Davis Co., 1903.

______, *The Sinusoidal Current as a Curative Agent,* Battle Creek, Michigan: The Good Health Publishing Co., 1913.

King, Lloyd E., Jr., "Brown Recluse Spider Bites: Stay Cool," *Journal of the American Medicial Association,* 54 (20): 2895-2896, November 22, 1985.

Kneipp, Sebastian, *The Codicil to "My Will for the Healthy and the Sick,"* Kempten, Bavaria: Koesel, 1897.

______, *My Water-Cure,* London: William Blackwood and Sons, 1893.

______, *My Will: A Legacy to the Healthy and the Sick,* Kempsten, Bavaria: Koesel, 1897.

Kovacs, Richard, *Electrotherapy and Light Therapy, With Essentials of Hydrotherapy and Mechanotherapy,* Philadelphia: Lea and Febiger, 1949.

Legan, Marshal Scott, "Hydropathy in America: A Nineteenth Century Panacea," *Bulletin of the History of Medicine,* (1): 267-280, Jan.-Feb., 1971.

Licht, Sidney, ed., *Medical Hydrology,* New Haven: Elizabeth Licht, 1963.

______, ed., *Therapeutic Heat and Cold,* Baltimore: Waverly Press, 1965.

Lindlahr, Henry, *Natural Therapeutics, Practice,* J. C. P. Proby, ed., Saffron Walden: C. W. Daniel Co., 1981.

______, *Nature Cure,* Chicago: The Nature Cure Publishing Co., 1922.

McKie, William L., *Scientific Hydrotherapy,* Sacramento: Dr. William L. McKie, 1957.

Moor, Fred B., et al., *Manual of Hydrotherapy and Massage,* Mountain View, California: Pacific Press Publishing Association, 1964.

Prentice, William E., *Therapeutic Modalities in Sports Medicine,* St. Louis: Times Mirror/Mosby College Publishing, 1986.

Price, Robin, "Hydropathy in England, 1840-1870," *Medical History,* 25: 269-280, 1981.

Rausse, J. H., *The Water-Cure Applied to Every Known Disease,* New York: Fowlers and Wells, 1858.

Rothschuh, Von Karl Eduard, "Die Konzeptualisierung der Naturheilkunde im 19. Jahrhundert," *Gesnerus,* 38 (1-2): 175-90, 1981.

Rothwieler, Ella L., et al., *The Art and Science of Nursing,* Philadelphia: F. A. Davis Co., 1954.

Schwartz, Gloria and Joe Coletto, "Herbal Hydrotherapeutics," on file National College of Naturopathic Medicine Library, Portland, Oregon, 1982.

Scott, Leo, *You Can Help Yourself to Health,* Spokane, Washington: Leo M. Scott, N.D., 1980.

Shew, Joel, *The Hydropathic Family Physician,* New York: Fowlers and Wells, 1856.

______, *Hydropathy, or the Water Cure,* New York: Fowlers and Wells, 1850.

______, *The Water-Cure Manual,* New York: Fowlers and Wells, 1849.

Sihler, Chr., *The Hydriatic Treatment of Typhoid Fever According to Brand, Tripier and Bouveret, and Bogel,* Cleveland: Published by Chr. Sihler, 1891.

Steele, Katharine McLean, *Psychiatric Nursing,* Philadelphia: F. A. Davis, Co., 4th edition, 1950.

Swannell, A. J., et al., "Changes in Arterial Blood Pressure in Patients Undergoing Routine Pool Therapy," *Physiotherapy,* 62 (3): 86-88, March, 1976.

Swinton, William E., "The Hydrotherapy and Infamy of Dr. James Gully," *Canadian Medical Association Journal,* 123: 1262-1264, December 20, 1980.

Szekely, Edmond Bordeaux, *Healing Waters,* San Diego: Academy Books, 1973.

Thrash, Agatha and Calvin, *Home Remedies, Hydrotherapy, Massage, Charcoal, and Other Simple Treatments,* Seale, Alabama: Yuchi Pines Institute Health Education Department, 1981.

Thomas, Charles, et al., *Simple Water Treatments for the Home,* Loma Linda, California: University Press, 1982.

Trall, R. T., *Hand-Book of Hygienic Practice,* Miller and Wood, Publishers, 1865.

______, *The Hydropathic Encyclopedia: A System of Hydropathy and Hygiene in Eight Parts,* New York: Fowlers and Wells, 1857.

Weiss, Harry B. and Howard R. Kemble, *The Great American Water-Cure Craze: A History of Hydropathy in the United States,* Trenton, New Jersey: The Past Times Press, 1967.

Wesselhoeft, Robert, et al., *The Water Cure in America, Over Three Hundred Cases of Various Diseases Treated with Water,* New York: Fowlers and Wells, Publishers, 1852.

Wright, Rebekah, *Hydrotherapy in Hosptials for Mental Diseases,* Boston: Tudor Press Inc., 1932.

INDEX

A New Lease on Life, 169
abdominal compress, 49, 80, 81, 194, 199, 202
ablution, 19, 49, 129
abscess, 117, 155, 199
acetaminophen, 56
acid burns, 165
Achillea, 165
Aconite, 192, 196, 197, 198
activated charcoal, 104, 115, 206
acupuncture, 3, 4, 24, 189, 206
Aesculus, 200
affusion, 19, 49, 59, 60, 107
alcohol rub, 70
alcoholism, 75, 122, 127, 131
alkali burns, 163
Allium cepa, 198
allopathic, 207
Aloes socotrina 157
alternate, 21, 41, 47, 111-113, 194, 197, 199, 200, 202
Althea, 165
Amaranthus, 160
amenorrhea, 161
American Hydropathic Institute, 11
American Magazine of Homeopathy and Hydropathy, 11
American Naturopathic Association, 12
Ammonium mur, 202
analgesic, 42
anemia, 76, 122, 127, 131
angina, 159, 196
ankle sprain, 49
anorexia, 54, 101, 131, 179
Anthracinum, 199
antibiotics, 54, 178
antibody, 54, 55
anticonvulsants, 57
Antimonium tart, 192
antipyretic, 56, 59
anxiety, 97, 127, 142, 147, 180, 193
Apis, 194, 196, 197, 200
appendicitis, 80, 101, 155, 182, 194, 195
Aralia, 160, 161
Arctostaphylos, 161, 162, 165
argyrol, 163
Arnica, 160, 161, 198, 199, 202
aromatic oils, 83
arrhythmias, 147
Arrow Glass Co., 156
Arsenicum, 193, 194, 197, 199
Artemisia, 157-159, 165
arterial trunk reflex, 43, 46
arteriosclerosis, 71, 76, 97, 122
arthritis, 81, 93, 113, 144, 170, 200, 208-209
Asarum, 198
Asclepias, 165
asphyxia, 194
aspirin, 56, 181, 209, 218
asthma, 80, 101, 128, 143, 144, 158, 159, 168, 170, 193
athletic injuries, 201-202
auscultation, 147-151, 181
autoimmune disease, 170
backache, 80
balneology, 19
Bard, Samuel, 9
barefoot walking, 7, 209
Barosma, 165
Baruch, Simon, 3, 5, 8, 14, 15, 23, 24, 211
Bastyr, John, 13-15, 147, 180, 181, 202-203
Battle Creek Sanatorium, 8
Bayberry, 160, 201
bee stings, 117
Bell, John, 9, 15
Belladonna, 57, 190, 192, 195, 196, 198, 200
Belle, Beth Adele, 169
benign prostatic hypertrophy, 89
Berberis, 165, 197, 198
betadyne, 111, 112
biliary colic, 198
biliary stasis, 80
Bilz, F. E., 7
black salve, 164, 201
blacks, 9
blepharitis, 198
blitz guss, 119-122
blood glucose, 32, 33, 207-208
bloody nose, 39
blue cobalt light, 201
Bluggerman, N., 166
Boericke and Tafel, 200
boils, 81, 93, 164, 180
borborygmi, 150
bran bath, 60
Brand bath, 60-61, 131
Brattleboro Infirmary, 9
bronchitis, 80, 94, 127, 143, 180

INDEX

Brown, John, 10
Brown, Mary, 10
brown recluse spider bites, 101
brown salve, 163
bruises, 113, 163; *see also* contusions *and* ecchymoses
Bryonia, 191, 192, 195, 199, 200
Buchu, 160; *see also Barosma*
Buerger's disease, 71
Bulwar-Lytton, Edward, 135
burns, 165
bursitis, 100, 200
"C" capsules, 157
C-reactive protein, 54
cactus, 162
Cactus, 197
Calcarea carb, 202
Calendula, 111, 112
cancer, 54, 109, 113, 144, 171; *see also* malignancy
Cantharis, 197
cape aloes, 157-159
Capsella, 162, 165
Capsicum, 163, 165
Carbo veg, 192
cardiac asthma, 85
cardiac collapse, 93
cardiac weakness 97, 128, 162
Carroll, Bill, 14, 173
Carroll, O. G., vii, 13-14, 15, 25, 101, 123, 135, 138, 145, 147, 157, 159, 165, 167-169, 173, 178, 179, 182, 183, 202
carrot poultice, 190
Castile soap, 104
cataplasm, 20
catnip, 104
Caulophyllum, 203
Cayce, Edgar, 156, 200
celiac pulse, 149, 150, 151, 154, 180
cellulitis, 41, 81, 113, 143, 197
centipede bites, 101
cerebral congestion, 45, 70, 96, 101, 180
ceruloplasmin, 54
chamomile, 104; *see also Chamomilla*
Chamomilla, 190, 194, 199
Chelidonium, 162, 198
chest compress, 80
chicken pox, 56
chilblains, 113
chill(ed,y), 71, 81, 127, 128, 131, 140, 141, 208, 216
chills, 54
Chimaphila, 165,
Chionanthus, 162
chiropractic, 12, 177
Cimicifuga, 203
Cina, 194
cisterna chyli, 180
claustrophobia, 128
Cleveland Chiropractic College, 13
clyster, 20
cobalt light, 202
Coca pulse test, 167
coffee, 104, 115
coffee poultice, 198
cold compress, 70, 74, 77, 93, 123, 125, 127, 135, 189, 190, 191, 195, 196, 198, 199, 200
cold mitten friction, 49, 74, 75, 79, 91, 93, 94, 116, 127, 128, 129-131, 192, 209
colds, 75, 79, 80, 94, 109, 127, 128, 131, 141, 144, 159, 209
Coletto, Joe, 166
colic, 89, 90, 104, 193-194
collateral circulation, 42-43, 45
Collinsonia, 162, 200
Colocynthis, 194
coma, 131
complement, 54
compress, 20, 31, 49, 50, 52, 61, 66, 91, 115
congestive headache, 42, 48, 71, 75, 89
congestive heart failure, 85
conjunctivitis, 198
constipation, 80, 89, 121, 127, 159
constitutional hydrotherapy, vii, 13, 25, 50, 123, 128, 135-145, 147, 150, 153-155, 167, 173, 177, 178, 181, 182, 191, 192, 193, 196, 198, 199, 200, 201, 202, 206, 207, 208, 209, 211-218
contractures, 202
contusions, 100
convalescence, 127
cough, 80, 84, 163
Coulter, J. S., 77
counterirritation, 20, 116
crenology, 19
Cretagus, 162
Crohn's disease, 80, 127, 143, 150, 170
Cuprum, 196
Curiosities of Common Water . . . in Curing Cholera, Intemperance, and other Maladies, 9

Currie, James, 7, 15
Cushings disease, 109
cystitis, 89, 101, 144, 161, 197
cystocele, 89
cytotoxic test, 167
D'Adamo, James, 167
debility, 76, 81, 90, 122, 128
decongestant, 42
deep vein thrombosis, 71
dehydration, 56, 57
delerium, 61, 127
dental pain, 199
dental surgery, 101, 199
depletion, 21, 100
depression, 97, 127, 131, 144, 154, 180
derivation, 20, 42, 43, 44-46, 50, 70, 89, 93, 126
dermatitis, 78
detoxification, 18, 36, 56, 62, 75, 101, 126, 127, 135, 138, 167, 175-185, 188, 205-206
diabetes, 7, 12, 57, 71, 76, 94, 96, 109, 113, 128, 144, 168, 185, 207-208
diabetic leg ulcers, 43, 143, 155
Diagnosis from the Eye, 13
diaphoretic, 74, 127, 192
diarrhea, 57, 80, 104, 179
diathermy (short wave), 142, 144, 151, 153-155, 190, 191, 192, 201
Dick, Harold, 14, 15, 17, 52, 101, 135, 145, 147, 148, 157, 159, 166, 173, 178, 181, 183, 184, 191, 195, 196, 202, 206, 207, 208 211
Dick, Ruby, 179
Dioscorea, 165, 198
diptheria, 11
disease crisis, 176, 180
Diseases of the Lungs, 193
douche, 7, 20, 39, 49, 119-122
drowning, 194
drug addiction, 122, 127, 185
drug intoxication, 75, 104
drug withdrawal, 97, 131
dry pack, 191
Dryopteris, 165
Dupuytren's contracture, 202
dwarf elder, 160, 161; *see also Aralia*
dysmenorrhea, 93, 144, 161
dyspepsia, 121, 143, 159
ecchymoses, 202
Echinacea, 162, 164, 165, 191, 197
eczema, 97, 107, 207
edema, 97, 113, 160
Egyptian oil, 200
Eizyaga, Francisco, 176
elder, 160, *see also Sambucus*
electrotherapy, 10, 128, 153-156
emaciation, 76
empiric, 5
encephalitis, 56
endogenous pyrogen, 53
enema, 103-105, 182, 188, 195
enuresis, 89, 160
epilepsy, 57, 109, 127
Epitome of Hydrotherapy, 8, 211
Epsom salts, 107, 108, 192, 197, 199, 200, 208
Equisetum, 160, 161, 197
Erdman, Frederick, 41
Errors of Physicians and Others in the Practice of Water Cure, 6
"Essay on the External Use of Water," 7
eucalyptus, 83
Eupatorium, 191
  perfoliatum, 165
  purpureum, 165
Euphrasia, 198
exhaustion, 194
exogenous pyrogen, 53
eye baths, 166
Farraday, cage of, 156
fasting, 56, 57, 62, 177, 181-184, 187, 188, 190, 191, 192, 199, 200, 206, 208, 209
fasting, dry, 6, 182, 194
fatigue, 71, 168, 171, 209, 217
Federal Communications Commission, 156
Ferrum phos, 192, 201
fever, 7, 19, 53-62, 81, 96, 97, 101, 103, 127, 131, 142, 144, 147, 155, 179, 182, 186, 189, 190, 192, 200, 217
fibrinogen, 54
fissures, 89
"5-5," 142, 143
"50" capsules, 158
flatulence, 179
Fleury, Louis, 5, 15
"flip," 138, 139, 140, 143, 189
Floyer, John, 5, 7, 9, 15
flu, 56, 75, 80, 127, 128, 131, 144, 191
fluxion, 21
fomentations, 20, 50, 66, 91-94, 131, 194, 198, 202
food intolerance, 167-173, 184, 206, 207, 208

food poisoning, 159, 194
foot tub, 66, 69
"⅘," 141, 143, 192, 208
"42" cocktail, 159, 194, 196
"42's," 159, 189, 191, 192, 194
fractures, 143
Francke, H., 6
friction, 49, 51, 56, 58-62, 107, 129-131, 192
friction mitts, 66
full-body bath, 45, 48, 60, 95, 189, 196, 198
"G" capsules, 158
gallbladder, 147
gallic acid, 164
gallstones, 93, 198
galvanism, 153, 200
Garrison, William Lloyd, 10
gastric ulcer, 94
gastritis, 122
gastroenteritis, 94
Gatchell, H.P., 10, 15, 193
gate theory, 49
Gelsemium, 191, 199
gentian, 157-158, 162, 165
ginger, 74, 165; *see also Zingiber*
glandulars, 189, 190
glaucoma, 198
glomerulonephritis, 197
goiter, 100
golden seal, 104, *see also Hydrastis*
gooseflesh, 52
gout, 6, 75
graduated bath, 60
Graefenberg, 5, 9, 10
Graham, Sylvester, 10
GTF chromium, 208
Guaiacum, 209
Gully, James, 7, 15
Hahn, Johann S., 5, 9, 15
Hahnemann, Samuel, 9, 15, 206
hallucinations, 180
Hamamelis, 165, 200
haptoglobulins, 54
headache, 100, 127, 143, 154, 170, 171, 180; *see also* congestive headache
healing crisis, 51, 97, 128, 142, 175-186, 187, 216, 218
heart disease, 76, 90, 122
heart drops, 162, 197
heart failure, 169; *see also* cardiac collapse
heat stroke, 53
heating compress, 20, 50, 77-81, 116, 123, 162, 189, 192, 193, 194, 197, 199, 208
heating pad, 23, 197
Helleborus, 196
hemorrhage, 44, 90, 94, 100, 160, 161, 200-201
hemorrhoids, 89, 101, 113, 144, 180, 200
Hepar sulph, 191
hepatic torpor, 80, 121, 162
hepatitis, 122
"Herbal Hydrotherapeutics," 166
Herbal Medication, A Clinical and Dispensatory Handbook, 165
herbs, 7, 115, 157-166, 189, 206
high frequency, 142, 144, 151, 154-156; *see also* Vita-ray
Hippocrates, 55, 56, 181
homeopathy, 3, 4, 9, 10, 24, 48, 57, 166, 176, 181, 182, 190, 206, 209
hopelessness, 180
horsetail, 165; *see also Equisetum* and rush
Hosack, David, 9
hot compress, 198, 199
hot evaporating sheet, 61
hot flash, 162
hot foot bath, 42, 45, 47, 48, 69-71, 73, 74, 75, 78, 89, 90, 91, 92, 93, 94, 107, 108, 109, 123, 189, 194, 200
hot tub, 27, 65, 209
hot water bottle, 92, 125, 197
Hydrastis, 165, 191
hydroculation, 91, 125
hydrogen peroxide, 111, 112
Hydropathic Encyclopedia, 10
hydropathy, 9-12, 19
Hygeio-Therapeutic College, 10
Hygeio-Therapy, 10
hygiene, 177
Hyoscyamus, 57, 196
Hypericum, 111, 112, 197, 199, 200
hypersensitivity, 144
hypertension, 76, 97, 144, 168, 170, 198-199
hyperthermia, 53, 54, 56
hyperthyroidism, 122, 147
hypoglycemic crisis, 208
hypopepsia, 121
hypotension, 75, 122
hypothalamus, 53, 54
hypothyroidism, 122
hysteria, 127
ice collar, 100, 101
ice pack, 9, 25, 42, 44, 45, 99-101, 194, 198 201, 202

ichthyol, 164
impaction, 104, 150
incontinence, 89
indigestion, 109, 127
infection, 53, 57, 62, 111, 112, 113, 117, 131 144, 164, 170, 188, 196-197
infertility, 144, 202
Influenzinum, 191
infrared 23, 124, 125, 188, 189, 197, 199
ingrown toenails, 113
insect bites, 101, 117
insomnia, 75, 80, 89, 93, 96, 97
insulin, 185, 207-208
intercostal neuralgia, 93
interferon, 54
interleukin-1, 53, 54
intrinsic, 30-32, 37, 39
Ipecac, 192, 193, 201
iridology, 13, 178-179, 183
Iris, 195
iritis, 198
irregular, 8, 9
irritable bowel syndrome, 80, 127, 143, 150
itching, 97
Jackson, James Caleb, 11, 15, 123, 176, 187, 205
jacuzzi, 131
jaundice, 75, 127, 180
Jensen Bernard, 178, 180
John Bastyr College, vii
Jones, Eli G., 108
Just, Adolphe, 7, 15
juvenile arthritis, 13
Kali bichromium, 191
Kali carb, 193
Kali mur, 190
Kali sulph, 191
Kalmia, 209
Kaltenleutgeben, 8
Kellogg, John Harvey, 8, 9, 10, 11, 13, 14, 15, 37, 109, 119, 154, 176, 177, 191, 201, 219
Kent, John T., 176, 196
kidney disease, 109, 155
kidney stones, 198
kinins, 188
Kluger, 55
Kneipp, Sebastian, 7, 12, 13, 14, 15, 119, 159, 165, 177
Kneipp Vademecum, 166
Kovacs, Richard, 65
Kreosotum, 194
Kuhne, Louis, 7, 15
Lac canium, 191
Lachesis, 190, 197
Lahn, Henry, 13, 15
lanolin, 96
laryngitis, 81, 84
lassitude, 61
latent heat, 25
Latrodectus, 197
LeDoux, Alex, 13, 15
LeDoux Institute of Natural Therapy, 13
Ledum, 198, 202
Leonorus, 156, 160
leopard's bane, 160, 161; *see also Arnica*
Lindlahr, Henry, 11-12, 13, 14, 15, 119, 167, 175, 176, 177, 180, 192, 205
liver congestion, 127; *see also* hepatic torpor
Lobelia, 193
Longfellow, Henry Wadsworth, 9
loofa, 129
lumbago, 89, 94
lung congestion, 141
Lust, Benedict, 11-12, 13, 14, 15
Lycopodium, 190, 191, 192, 197, 198, 209
lymphadenopathy, 81
lymphangitis, 81, 113, 144, 197
Mag mur, 198
Mag phos, 194
malabsorption, 127
malaria, 54
maldigestion, 80
malignancy, 55, 94, 104, 144
malposition, 202, 203
mania, 96, 127
manipulation, 93, 182, 189, 196, 202, 206
marjoram, 160, 161
Marrubium, 165
massage, 8, 12, 75, 93, 177, 189, 202, 206
mastitis, 80, 154
measles, 127
Medical Diagnosis, 147
melancholy, 127
meningitis, 56, 196
menopause, 161
menorrhagia, 89, 90
menstruation, suppressed, 71, 89
mental dullness, 170
mental illness, 95, 97
Mentha, 165
Merc. iod. flav., 191

Merc. iod. rub., 191
Merc. sol., 191
Mercurius, 191, 192,
Methodism, 7
migraine, 100
Millifollium, 201
Mitchella, 161
motherwort, 160; *see also Leonurus*
Mt. Carmel Orphan Asylum, 13
multiple sclerosis, 171
Muriatic acid, 200
muscle soreness, 93
muscle tension, 93
mustard plaster, 20
mustard poultice, 195-196
mustard powder, 69, 70, 91, 115, 189
My Water Cure, 7
myocardial infarction, 94, 148, 196
Myrica, 165
Nash, E. B., 193
National College of Naturopathic Medicine, vii, 14, 145, 166, 213, 216
Nat mur, 198, 200
Nat sulph, 196
Natural Healing Method, 7
nature cure, 7
Nature Cure, 12
nausea, 158, 179, 180, 184, 195-196, 202
Neo-Naturopathy, 7
nephritic colic, 89
nephritis, 94, 122, 127, 197
Nervine capsules, 158
nervous agitation, 75, 122, 127
nervous exhaustion, 97, 131
neuralgia, 89
neurasthenia, 109, 121, 127, 154
neutral bath, 48, 60, 62, 95-97, 107
Nichols, Mary Gove, 11
Nichols, Thomas Lowe, 11, 15
nicotine addiction, 127
non-ionized water, 138, 145
nosebleed, 39, 71, 200
nutrition, 167-173, 206
Nux Vomica, 57, 191, 192, 193, 194, 198, 200
obesity, 90, 127, 144
obstetrics, 202-203
Ocimum, 198
olive oil, 104
One Man's Food Is . . . Someone Else's Poison, 167
onion poultice, 202
Ontario College of Naturopathic Medicine, vii
Opium, 196
Oregon grape, 162; *see also Berberis*
Organon of Medicine, 206
orthodox medicine, 5, 8, 9, 24, 56
Oscillococcinum, 191
Osler, William, 56
otitis media, 171, 190
Our Home on the Hillside, 11
ovarian cysts, 201
ovaritis, 94
pain, 81, 93, 97, 100, 103, 104, 117, 155, 188, 189, 219
Pariera, 198
peanut oil, 109
pelvic congestion, 71, 89, 90, 141
pelvic inflammatory disease, 89, 201
peppermint, 163; *see also Mentha*
peripheral heart, 36, 42
peripheral vascular disease, 71, 76, 90, 94, 113
pharyngitis, 81
Phosphoric acid, 208
Phosphorus, 192, 208
physiological zero, 96
Physio-medicalist, 165
Physostygma, 198
Phytolacca, 190
pinworms, 104, 159
pipsissewa, 162, 164; *see also Chimaphila*
plantar warts, 71
pneumococcus, 54, 55
pneumonia, 80, 127, 180, 191
Podophyllum, 162, 174
poison, 75, 104
polio virus, 54
Populus, 165
Portland Naturopathic Clinic, 217
postpartum, 89, 160
potato poultice, 198
poultice, 20, 115-117
Prednisone, 209
pregnancy, 95, 97, 162, 202-203
Pregnancy tea, 161, 202
premenstrual syndrome, 143
Priessnitz of America, 10
Preissnitz, Vincent, 5-6, 7, 9, 10, 14, 15, 123, 124, 177
Priest, A. W., 165
Priest, L. R., 165

Primitive Physick, 7
Primum non nocere, 205
Principles and Practice of Hydrotherapy, 8
prolapsus, 89, 90
prophylaxis, 75
prostaglandin E_2, 53, 54
prostatitis, 89, 94, 200
pruritis ani, 89
pruritis valvae, 89
psoriasis, 144, 207
Psycho-Hygienic, 11
psyllium seed, 200
pulmonary congestion, 71; *see also* lung congestion
Pulsatilla, 190, 191, 192, 193, 197, 203, 209
Pulte, J. H., 10, 15
pyelonephritis, 197
pyridoxal alpha-ketoglutarate, 208
Pyrogenium, 194, 199
quassia bark, 104
RAST, 167
Rathanhia, 200
Rational Hydrotherapy, 8, 119, 219
Rausse, J. H., 6, 15, 175, 176, 177, 184
Raynaud's disease, 144
reactive, 30-32, 37, 39
rectocele, 89
red blood cells, 14, 32, 33, 131, 138
reflex areas, 37-39, 44-46, 48, 89, 92, 201
renal colic, 93, 198
renal failure, 104
respiratory congestion, 84, 90; *see also* lung congestion
respiratory infection, 171
Respiratory Leaders, 193
restlessness, 61, 127
retracings, 177
retrostasis, 21, 42, 43, 45, 49, 100
Return to Nature, 7
revulsive, 21, 41, 45, 47, 197
Reye's syndrome, 56
Rheum, 194
rheumatic diathesis, 141, 170, 208
rheumatic fever, 9, 13
rheumatism, 6, 50, 93, 122
rheumatoid arthritis, 75, 112, 209
Rhododendron, 209
rhubarb, 163
Rhus tox, 202, 209
Romberg, Moritz, 35
Rouge, Father, 13, 15
roundworms, 159
Ruggles, David, 9-10, 15
rush, 160, 161; *see also Equisetum*
Rush, Benjamin, 9, 15
Russian bath, 26, 69, 73-76, 122, 131
Ruta, 200, 202
salicylates, 55
salt glow, 107-109
Sambucus, 160
Sarsaparilla, 197
sauna, 27, 53, 131, 177, 191
scarlet fever, 127
Schroth, Johann, 6, 15
Schwartz, Gloria, 166
sciatica, 89, 94, 122
Scott, D. J., 184
Scott, Leo, 14, 15, 101, 143, 145, 147, 165, 169, 181
Scutellaria, 158, 165
seizures, 57
sensory loss, 71, 94, 113
Sepia, 200
Seventh Day Adventism, 11
sexual excitement, 89
Shelton, Herbert, 56, 184
shepherd's purse, 162; *see also Capsella*
Shew, Joel, 10, 11, 15
Shew, Mary Louis, 10
Shivering, 53, 58, 59, 61, 62
Silicea, 191, 200
sine wave, 8, 136-144, 150, 151, 153-154, 196, 202, 208, 213
sinus congestion, 75, 127
sinusitis, 170, 191
sitz bath, 12, 47, 48, 66, 87-90, 197, 202
skin heart, 36
skullcap, 157-158; *see also Scutellaria*
smallpox, 5
Smith, John, 9, 15
Smollet, Tobias, 7
sore throat, 84, 190
spasm, 89, 90, 202
spasmodic breathing, 84
Special "G", 158
specific gravity, urine, 185
specific heat, 25-27
Speisman pack, 192
spirochetes, 54
spleen, 121
spondylotherapy, 189, 198
sponge bath, 61

sprains, 81, 93, 100, 113, 163, 202
squaw vine, 161; *see also Mitchella*
stage fright, 89
steam baths, 53
steam inhalation, 83-85
Sticta, 200
stings, 164
St. Johnswort, 160; *see also Hypericum*
stone root, 162
Stowe, Harriet Beecher, 9
strain, 113
Strammonium, 57, 196
stroke, 101
Strontium carb, 202
stupe, 20
sublingual test, 167
suffocation, 194
Sulphur, 192, 200
sunbathing, 53
sunburn, 163
sweat baths, 6
Swedish movement, 10
Symphytum, 165, 198
syphilis, 54
tachycardia, 101
tannic acid, 163
Tarantula cub., 199
TB, 12
temperature conversions, 67-68
tenesmus, 89
tennis elbow, 100
Terebenthina, 197
thermometry, 7, 50, 66, 141
thermotherapy, 23, 27, 29, 53, 57, 59, 61
Thomsonian, 13
Thrash, Agatha and Calvin, 191
throat compress, 81, 190
thromboangiitis obliterans, 71
thyme, 165
thyrotropin-releasing factor, 53
Tilden, John H., 176
tobacco, 75, 131; *see also* nicotine
tongue diagnosis, 179-181
tonsilitis, 81
toothache, 100
toxemia of pregnancy, 95, 97
Traite-Pratique et Raisonne D'Hydrotherapie, 7
Trall, Russell Thatcher, 10, 15, 147, 175
Treatise on Baths, 9
trigger point therapy, 189
trunk compress, 49, 78, 80, 192, 194
Truth, Sojourner, 10
Tuberculinum, 191, 192
tumor pain, 198
tumors, 164, 168
turmeric, 163
typhoid, 60
ulcerative colitis, 80, 104, 127, 143, 150, 176
ultraviolet, 188, 189
umbilical compress, 49, 193
Underground Railroad, 9
unorthodox, 5
urinary tract infection, 89, 90; *see also* cystitis
uterine fibroids, 201
uterine hemorrhage, 200
uterine prolapse, 89
uva ursi, 161, 162, 168; *see also Arctostaphylos*
vaginal pack, 201
vaginismus, 89
vaginitis, 89
valerian, 157-158, 165
vaporizers, 83
varicose veins, 144, 162, 202, 209
venous stasis ulcers, 113
Veratrum, 194
vertigo, 127
Viburnum, 165
vinegar, 111, 112, 198
visceral manipulation, 75
Vis Medicatrix Naturae, 54, 55, 206
Vita-ray, 156, 190, 199
Vithoulkas, George, 176
vomiting, 57, 179, 195-196
water cure, 6, 7, 8, 9-12, 19
Water Cure Applied to Every Known Disease, 6
Water Cure for Ladies, 10
Water Cure in Chronic Disease, 7
Water Cure Journal, 10
Water Cure Manual, 10
weakness, 76, 109, 127, 131
Wesley, John, 7
Wesselhoeft, Robert, 9-10, 11, 15
Wesselhoeft, William, 9-10, 11
wet sheet pack, 26, 123-128, 131, 182, 191, 192, 196, 197, 200
whirlpools, 65
white blood cells, 18, 32, 33, 54, 131, 138
White, Ellen, G., 11, 15

white oak bark, 164, 165
white salve, 164
Winternitz, Wilhelm, 8, 9, 14, 15
witch hazel, 70, 162, 163, 174, 200; *see also Hamamelis*
women's health, 11
women's rights, 11
wormwood, 157-159; *see also Artemisia*
yarrow, 191; *see also Achillea*
Yates County *Chronicle,* 11
"You Can Help Yourself to Health," 165
zinc oxide, 163, 164
Zincum, 196
Zingiber, 165

ABOUT THE AUTHORS

Dr. Boyle is a graduate of the National College of Naturopathic Medicine in Portland, Oregon. He has taught at National College and at the Canadian College of Naturopathic Medicine in Toronto. Besides maintaining a private practice, he is also a continuing education instructor for the American Association of Naturopathic Physicians, and is on the faculty of Southwest College of Naturopathic Medicine and Health Sciences.

Dr. Saine is also a graduate of National College. He is a Diplomate of the Homeopathic Academy of Naturopathic Physicians. He is founder and dean of the Canadian Academy of Homeopathy. He is on the faculty of the National Center for Homeopathy Summer School and has lectured widely in the fields of homeopathic and naturopathic medicine. He is in private practice in Toronto and Montreal.

OTHER TITLES FROM BUCKEYE NATUROPATHIC PRESS

Herb Doctors: Pioneers in Nineteenth-Century American Botanical Medicine, by Wade Boyle, N.D., 1988.

Reading the Eye, Pulse and Tongue for the Indicated Remedy, by Eli G. Jones, M.D., 1989.

Official Herbs: Botanical Substances in the United States Pharmacopoeias, 1820-1990, by Wade Boyle, N.D., 1991.

Fasting: Signs and Symptoms, A Clinical Guide, by Trevor K. Salloum, N.D., 1991.